PEDIATRIC AND NEONATAL SURGERY

Edited by **Joanne Baerg**

Pediatric and Neonatal Surgery
http://dx.doi.org/10.5772/63041
Edited by Joanne Baerg

Contributors

Esra Caliskan, Abdulkerim Temiz, Eva Miranda Marwali, Nikolaus Haas, Beatrice Heineking, Marissa Vadi, Chelan Nour, Harmony Carter, Patrick Leiter, Shelly Haug, Anamika Banerji, Sara Farooqi, Andrew Hopper, Kenneth Gow

Published by InTech

Janeza Trdine 9, 51000 Rijeka, Croatia

Publishing Process Manager Edi Lipovic
Technical Editor SPi Global
Cover InTech Design team

First published April, 2017
Printed in Croatia
Legal deposit, Croatia: National and University Library in Zagreb

Additional hard copies can be obtained from orders@intechopen.com

Pediatric and Neonatal Surgery, Edited by Joanne Baerg
p. cm.
Print ISBN 978-953-51-3135-9
Online ISBN 978-953-51-3136-6

For EU product safety concerns:
IN TECH d.o.o., Prolaz Marije Krucifikse Kozulić 3, 51000 Rijeka, Croatia,
info@intechopen.com or visit our website at intechopen.com.

Meet the editor

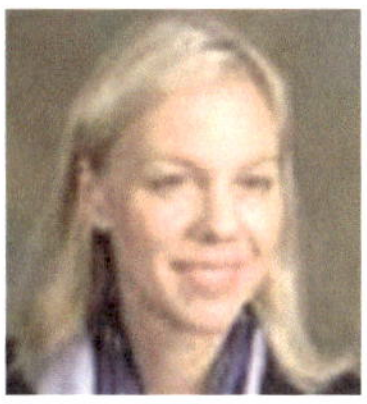

Dr. Joanne Baerg is an associate professor of Pediatric Surgery at Loma Linda University Children's Hospital. She has a specific interest in clinical research in pediatric surgery and is the director of the Pediatric Surgery Clinical Scholars Research Program. She is a member of the American Pediatric Surgery Association and the Surgical Section of the American Academy of Pediatrics.

Contents

Preface

Neonatal and Pediatric Surgery is a broad field with many challenges. The aim of this short book is to provide the reader with several chapters in the field of neonatal and pediatric surgery. Each chapter provides details on a specific area of this changing field. The scope of this book focuses on a few areas that are rare and challenging. For example, it covers preoperative and postoperative care of neonates. Important anesthesia considerations, including anesthesia for neonates and regional anesthesia, are discussed. A unique chapter on neonatal tumors is presented. The book provides an overview of the recent recommendations for care of infants and children that undergo cardiac surgery. The challenging aspects of caustic ingestion are explained.

Each chapter stands alone as a detailed source of information for the reader. This book brings updated information with structured headings that will allow the reader to remain focused as the material is reviewed. I would like to thank all the authors that contributed their time and expertise to this project.

Joanne E. Baerg MD, FACS
Loma Linda University Children's Hospital
Loma Linda, CA, USA

Section 1

Peri-Operative Care of the Neonate

Chapter 1

Perioperative Care of the Neonate

Shelly Haug, Sara Farooqi, Anamika Banerji and
Andrew Hopper

Additional information is available at the end of the chapter

http://dx.doi.org/10.5772/67174

Abstract

Care of the perioperative neonate requires careful consideration of many aspects including the impact of anesthesia and surgery on multiple organ systems. Neonatal care should include close attention to achieving homeostasis and stability in the perioperative period. This chapter will address the critical elements in the management of the surgical neonate.

Keywords: neonate, surgical care, Neonatal Intensive Care Unit (NICU)

1. Preoperative care of the neonate

Care of the preoperative surgical neonate starts with a comprehensive history and physical examination on admission. It is important to focus on airway, respiratory, cardiac, and renal abnormalities which may impact surgery. Preoperative lab studies should include a complete blood count with differential, basic metabolic panel, coagulation studies and cross match blood screening [1, 2].

Preoperative airway management includes consideration of need for intubation and mechanical ventilation and chest radiography to confirm endotracheal tube position, to assess lung volumes and to evaluate cardiomegaly. Endotracheal intubation is often completed by the neonatal intensive care physician though at times pediatric anesthesia may prefer this responsibility; therefore, communication is important.

Additional preoperative goals include optimizing ventilation and oxygenation, correcting abnormal electrolytes and pH and ensuring adequate perfusion. Lab work should forewarn clinicians of anemia and thrombocytopenia which should be corrected with goal neonatal hematocrit of 30–35% and platelet count greater than 100,000 preoperatively. Coagulation studies should be normalized with fresh frozen plasma and cryoprecipitate as needed prior to surgery. In cases of liver dysfunction, consider vitamin K administration. Disseminated intravascular coagulation should be considered and treated if sepsis is suspected. Ideally, surgery should be deferred if sepsis is suspected.

Adequate intravenous access is necessary prior to surgery. The need for central venous line placement should be determined and discussed with the anesthesiologist and pediatric surgeon in advance. If percutaneous central venous line placement is unsuccessful, central venous line may need to be placed by surgery. Factors that should be weighed in determining the need for central line placement include type of surgery, anticipated recovery time and anticipated length of time to regain bowel function. If the neonate is expected not to tolerate adequate enteral volumes for appropriate nutrition or to be nil per os (NPO) for greater than 2 – 5 days, then central line access should be considered [3].

Length of NPO status should be discussed with the surgeon. For elective procedures requiring anesthesia or sedation, the American Society of Anesthesiologists recommends neonates be NPO for at least 4 hours if fed breast milk and 6 hours if fed formula prior to surgery [4]. NPO status is at times outweighed by the need for emergency surgery in cases of critical illness.

Choice of intravenous fluid replacement is in large part dictated by the disease process, surgery and type of therapy anticipated [5]. Intravenous fluids should include provision for maintenance fluids and, if indicated, fluid and electrolyte replacement to correct deficits and for surgical conditions with anticipated fluid loss (see **Table 1**). Neonates are born with excess total body water in comparison with muscle mass and fat. The more preterm neonates have increased extracellular fluid. After birth, there is a shift of fluid from the extracellular compartment that results in salt and water diuresis by 48 to 72 hours and physiological weight loss in the first week of life. Failure to have adequate diuresis is associated with increased morbidities including pulmonary edema, tissue edema, symptomatic patent ductus arteriosus, necrotizing enterocolitis (NEC) and chronic lung disease [5–8]. Neonates are more sensitive to hypovolemia due to relatively low cardiac contractility. Maintenance fluid replacement should allow for the initial loss of extracellular fluid diuresis over the first week of life while maintaining normal intravascular volume and tonicity reflected by heart rate, urine output, electrolytes and acid/base status [5].

Birth weight (g)	Insensible water loss (mL/kg/day)	Total water requirement by age (mL/kg/day)		
		Day 1–2	Day 3–7	Day 8–30
<750	100+	100–200	120–200	120–180
750–1000	60–70	80–150	100–150	120–180
1001–1500	30–65	60–100	80–150	120–180
>1500	15–30	60–80	100–150	120–180

Adapted from Ref. [45].

Table 1. Maintenance fluid requirements during the first month of life [5].

Careful estimation of ongoing pathogenic fluid losses is important to determine the best volume and composition of fluid replacement. Estimation of fluid and electrolyte losses can be difficult especially in conditions that predispose to third spacing such as sepsis, hypoalbuminemia, intra-abdominal infection, postoperative abdominal surgery or cardiac surgery. Calculating daily gross intake and output along with serial weight can help to estimate fluid loss. Electrolyte losses can be estimated by multiplying the volume of fluid loss by the electrolyte content of the type of body fluid (see **Table 2**) [5].

Fluid source	**Sodium (mmol/L)**	**Potassium (mmol/L)**	**Chloride (mmol/L)**
Stomach	20–80	5–20	100–150
Small intestine	100–140	5–15	90–120
Bile	120–140	5–15	90–120
Ileostomy	45–135	3–15	20–120
Diarrheal stool	10–90	10–80	10–110
Adapted from Ref. [45].			

Table 2. Electrolyte content of body fluids [5].

Normal saline boluses of 10–20 mL/kg should be given to maintain adequate renal perfusion to ensure normal urine output (2–3 mL/kg/hour). Fluid should also be given to maintain normal blood pressure based on gestational age. Caution should be used when administering greater than 40 mL/kg of fluid boluses to support blood pressure as this should prompt evaluation regarding the cause of hypotension. Fluid boluses must be balanced by the risk of patent ductus arteriosus in at-risk preterm neonates. Need to increase total fluid intake may be better tolerated by gradually increasing overall total daily fluid rate rather than by giving fluid boluses. Metabolic acidosis can be buffered by the administration of sodium acetate in fluids given to maintain central line patency. Hypoproteinemia should be corrected slowly if possible preoperatively to ensure better postoperative wound healing. An early assessment of serum albumin should be considered, as this may be reflective of prognosis for severity of gastroschisis. In most instances, administration of albumin for fluid replacement and to correct hypoalbuminemia should be discouraged as the albumin leaks into the tissues and contributes to tissue edema. Consideration should be given to placement of a Foley catheter for very long procedures or very unstable or chemically paralyzed neonates. Perfusion should be monitored and normalized. Assessment of tissue perfusion includes measuring blood pressure by peripheral cuff or by arterial line placement. Monitoring arterial blood pressure by indwelling arterial line is indicated for critically ill neonates if a period of postoperative instability is expected, if the neonate is requiring vasopressors or for frequent blood sampling.

Significant morbidity and mortality of perioperative neonates are related to hypoxic/ischemic events. Most intensive care units monitor perfusion index as part of skin surface oxygen saturation monitoring [9, 10]. More institutions are using near infrared spectroscopy (NIRS) to assess tissue perfusion. While pulse oximetry provides a measure of arterial oxygen saturation, it may not be particularly useful for determining oxygen delivery to the tissues. NIRS regional oximetry measures the balance between local oxygen delivery and consumption beneath the sensor. NIRS provides an end-organ measure of not only oxygenation, but also perfusion. NIRS can be used as a continuous, real-time, noninvasive bedside monitor using infrared light sensors of regional tissue oxygenation and hemodynamics [11]. It is United States Food and Drug Administration (FDA) approved for use in neonates, including those less than 2.5 kg. Regional tissue oxygen saturation reflects a ratio of arterial and venous blood (25:75%) and the balance between oxygen delivery and tissue consumption. NIRS monitoring usually includes measuring cerebral and somatic, either renal or mesenteric, regional oxygen saturation. There are norms of average NIRS values for cerebral, renal and mesenteric areas of monitoring, providing a noninvasive measure of end-organ oxygenation and perfusion [12]. These norms vary between term and preterm neonates (see **Table 3**).

rSO2	Term	Preterm
Cerebral (%)	66–89	66–83
Renal (%)	75–97	64–87
Mesenteric (%)	63–87	32–66

Values differ by sensor type with neonatal sensors reading 10% higher. Adapted from Refs. [13, 14].

Table 3. Normal ranges of regional oxygen saturation (rSO2) in term [13] and preterm [14] neonates.

Gastric decompression by Replogle sump tube should be discussed with surgeon and must be considered for neonates with intestinal obstruction. Cases to strongly consider gastric decompression include surgical necrotizing enterocolitis, Hirschsprung's disease, intestinal atresias, gastroschisis and omphalocele.

Preoperative labs should be obtained within 24 hours of planned surgery to ensure infection is ruled out. Prophylactic antibiotics should be given within 1 hour of skin entry [1]. At some hospitals, this timing is best achieved if antibiotic such as cefazolin is given in the preoperative surgical area as part of a preoperative checklist. Antibiotic choice should be dependent on disease process. Suspected perforation should be treated with broad-spectrum antibiotics that specifically include Gram-negative and anaerobic coverage. Length of therapy and choice of antibiotics may change depending on the intraoperative findings and culture results.

2. Common conditions of the surgical neonate

Although various conditions require specific management, the initial management of the surgical neonate consists of gastric decompression with placement of a Replogle tube, imaging including abdominal radiographs, and fluid and electrolyte management. The use of antibiotics is dependent upon the suspected pathology. Specialized management considerations are reviewed for the following conditions.

2.1. Gastroschisis

Gastroschisis is a congenital anterior abdominal wall defect that occurs to the right of the umbilical cord insertion that results in herniation of abdominal contents and thereby permitting bowel exposure to amniotic fluid in utero [15]. Abdominal contents generally contain the small intestine; however, larger defects may contain the stomach and colon [16]. Compared to an omphalocele defect, there is no transparent sac to protect the intestine and gastroschisis is not usually associated with other congenital syndromes. However, it may be associated with other gastrointestinal abnormalities such as malrotation, atresia or stenosis. A neonate with a prenatal diagnosis of gastroschisis should preferably be delivered at an institution with multidisciplinary care, influx into maternal-fetal medicine service, neonatal intensive care team and pediatric surgery. At the time of delivery, the neonate should be placed in a bowel bag enclosed to the neonate's axilla. This bag protects the bowel and also helps to retain body heat. Given the location of the defect, the neonate should be placed right side down to avoid tension on the mesenteric vasculature. A Replogle tube should be placed at the time of delivery to allow for abdominal decompression. All neonates should receive empiric broad-spectrum antibiotics, preferably ampicillin and gentamicin. Immediate intubation is not required if the neonate's respiratory status is stable. Some medical experts recommend a controlled, elective intubation to avoid unnecessary airway trauma. Surgical management is dependent on the defect. Surgical options include primary closure, staged reduction with a silo or sutureless umbilical closure [17]. In order to prepare the neonate for surgery, a secure airway should be established as well as adequate intravenous access. Due to the nature of the defect, umbilical lines are contraindicated in gastroschisis. Chemical paralysis is generally dependent on the preference of the surgeon and may be required in neonates with a large defect. When defect size or abdominal pressure issues prevent primary closure, placement of a silo allows for gradual reduction in the intestine into the abdominal cavity. With a silo, abdominal contents are gently "squeezed" into the abdomen daily. Once the contents are reduced, the neonate is taken to the operating room for closure. After the defect is closed, nasogastric decompression is continued until return of bowel function.

Special consideration must be taken in regard to fluid management in gastroschisis due to insensible fluid loss and postoperative third-space fluid shifts. Amount of postoperative fluid administration should generally be less than prior to gastroschisis closure and be balanced with perfusion and urine output [18]. See discussion of preoperative fluid management. Potential complications associated with gastroschisis include ileus, sepsis, intestinal atresias, malabsorption, wound infection and necrotizing enterocolitis [16].

2.2. Omphalocele

An omphalocele is a congenital ventral abdominal wall defect of the umbilical ring that results in abdominal viscera herniation and is associated with chromosomal, cardiac and/or genitourinary abnormalities [19]. Immediate postnatal management should include protection of the herniated viscera with sterile saline-soaked gauze, and stabilization of viscera to ensure blood supply to the bowel is not kinked by the weight of the bowel. The neonate may be placed right side down or with towels placed under the bowel to help support the externalized intestine.

Gastric decompression should be initiated with placement of a Replogle tube on continuous low suction to prevent bowel distention. If volume of gastric drainage exceeds approximately 10 mL/kg per 12 hour shift, gastric fluid should be replaced with 0.9% sodium chloride.

Potential problems with omphalocele include risk of hypothermia due to high heat loss from the exposed bowel as well as risk of vasoconstriction, decreased tissue perfusion and metabolic acidosis [19]. Fluids and electrolyte replacement will need to anticipate additional fluid losses due to the specific disease pathology. Maintenance of intravascular fluid volume is necessary to ensure adequate tissue perfusion and preservation of bowel wall perfusion [19, 20].

Other factors to consider include prevention of sepsis by administering broad-spectrum antibiotic therapy. Due to the association with other anomalies, neonates with omphalocele should be evaluated with chest and abdominal radiography, renal and abdominal ultrasound as well as echocardiogram prior to operation [19]. Repair of the defect will be a primary or a staged closure depending on the size of the defect. Potential postoperative complications include significant increase in intra-abdominal pressures that may compromise venous blood return and hemodynamic and/or respiratory stability due to diaphragmatic elevation [19].

Another important consideration in neonates with omphalocele is the risk of pulmonary hypertension [21]. All neonates with omphalocele should be monitored for evidence of pulmonary hypertension between the second and seventh day after birth as they may not initially present with signs of pulmonary hypertension. Diagnosis should be suspected based on increased oxygen requirement and increased pre- and postductal gradient and confirmed by increased right ventricular pressures (greater than 40 mmHg) on echocardiogram [21].

Short-term postoperative complications include necrotizing enterocolitis, prolonged ileus and respiratory distress. If primary closure is done, the neonate will require assisted ventilation and may require muscle relaxants for a time. It is important to ensure adequate ventilation and oxygenation by adjusting inspiratory and end expiratory pressures to maintain adequate lung volumes as the abdominal distention postoperatively may be aggravated by fluid third spacing due to capillary leak syndrome. Postoperative pain management usually requires continuous infusion of morphine and should be titrated according to appropriate neonatal pain scales (see pain section later in chapter) [22]. Long-term complications include prolonged dependence on parenteral nutrition, gastroesophageal reflux, parenteral nutrition-related liver disease, feeding intolerance and neurodevelopmental delay [19]. When bowel function returns postoperatively, initiation of enteral feeds should be done with breast milk or an elemental formula such as Elecare or Neocate, starting with small volumes and advancing slowly [23, 24]. Neonates with giant omphalocele usually require prolonged time to achieve full enteral feeds, especially if complicated by respiratory insufficiency requiring intubation shortly after delivery or symptoms of gastroesophageal reflux postoperatively [24].

2.3. Obstruction

See further detail (**Table 4**).

Type	Presentation	Diagnosis	Preoperative care	Treatment	Postoperative care
Duodenal atresia	Few hours after birth; bilious vomiting, no distention	Abdominal film; "double-bubble" sign	Gastric decompression, IV fluids	Diamond-shaped duodenoduodenostomy	Feeding dependent upon bowel function
Malrotation with volvulus	At 3–7 days; bilious vomiting, rapid deterioration with volvulus	Ultrasound and contrast studies; "upper GI spiral" sign, abnormal location of the superior mesenteric vessels	Gastric decompression, IV fluids, STAT surgery for symptomatic patients	Ladd's procedure	Feeding dependent upon bowel function
Jejunoileal atresia	Within 1 day of birth; vomiting, abdominal distention	Abdominal film; air-fluid levels	Gastric decompression, IV fluids	Resection and anastomosis	Feeding dependent upon bowel function
Meconium ileus	Immediately after birth; abdominal distention, bilious vomiting	Abdominal film; distention, air-fluid levels, "ground-glass" sign	Gastric decompression, IV fluids	Enterostomy if complicated; gastrografin enema	Acetylcysteine (Mucomyst), pancreatic enzymes
Necrotizing ileus	Varied timing; feeding intolerance, abdominal distention, vomiting, bloody stools	Serial abdominal films; distention, ileus, pneumatosis intestinalis, portal venous gas	Gastric decompression, IV fluids, antibiotics for 7 to14 days, serial imaging, STAT surgery if perforated	Resection of necrotic bowel and enterostomy	Feeding reinitiation with slow advancement after antibiotic course completion and normal imaging

Adapted from Ref. [25].

Table 4. Neonatal obstruction [25].

2.4. Necrotizing enterocolitis

Necrotizing enterocolitis (NEC) is the most common emergent neonatal gastrointestinal diseases among premature neonates [26]. The mortality rate of NEC may range from 20 to 30% with the highest mortality in those neonates who require surgery [27]. Often, an inverse relationship between gestational age and frequency of NEC exists. Therefore, the smaller the neonate, the higher the clinical suspicion for this disease.

Typically, NEC presents with feeding intolerance, hematochezia and abdominal distention. Clinical progression of the disease may ensue rapidly from abdominal discoloration, worsening distention with intestinal perforation leading to clinical deterioration with hypotension, metabolic acidosis and thrombocytopenia requiring intensive medical and surgical support. At the moment of suspicion for NEC, the neonate should be placed NPO and gastric decompression initiated. Intravenous fluid hydration must be provided, along with an urgent surgical consultation. Intravenous antibiotics should be started once NEC is suspected that often include "triple therapy" consisting of Gram-positive, Gram-negative and anaerobic bacteria coverage. Immediate and serial abdominal radiographs should be obtained to assess the presence of pneumatosis intestinalis, one of the hallmarks to diagnose NEC. Laboratory testing should include blood cultures, complete blood count (CBC) to assess for leukocytosis and thrombocytopenia, and C-reactive protein. Serial two-view abdominal radiographs should be obtained to assess for progression. While there are no universally accepted criteria for NEC, Bell's staging system is often used to describe the stages and severity of this disease. The staging is described as follows (see **Table 5**).

Stage/classification	Systemic signs	Abdominal signs	Radiographic signs
IA; suspected	Temperature instability, apnea, bradycardia, lethargy	Gastric residuals, abdominal distention, emesis, heme-positive stool	Normal or intestinal dilation, mild ileus
IB; suspected	Same as above	Gross hematochezia	Same as above
IIA; definite, mildly ill	Same as above	Same as above with absent bowel sounds with or without abdominal distention	Intestinal dilation, ileus, pneumatosis intestinalis
IIB definite, moderately ill	Same as above plus mild metabolic acidosis and thrombocytopenia	Same as above, plus absent bowel sounds, definite tenderness, with or without abdominal cellulitis or right lower quadrant mass	Same as IIA plus ascites
IIIA advanced, severely ill, intact bowel	Same as IIB plus hypotension, bradycardia, severe apnea, combined respiratory and metabolic acidosis, DIC and neutropenia	Same as above, plus signs of peritonitis, marked tenderness and abdominal distention	Same as IIA plus ascites
IIIB advanced, severely ill, perforated bowel	Same as IIIA	Same as IIIA	Same as above plus pneumoperitoneum

Adapted from Ref. [28].

Table 5. Modified Bell's staging criteria for necrotizing enterocolitis [28].

3. Comparison between acute and elective surgical management

Operative intervention of the acutely ill neonate is less desirable but often unavoidable. In situations of intestinal perforation or a hemodynamically compromised neonate, all efforts should be made to ensure a near stable status of the neonate [1, 2, 5]. If a neonate requires emergent surgical intervention, communication with the surgical team, anesthesiology and neonatology team to discuss diagnosis and planned intervention must be made as soon as possible. Most important in management is establishing a stable airway and adequate intravenous or central line access. Pertinent imaging including radiographs and ultrasound should be readily available for evaluation by the surgical team. The neonatal team should ideally be at bedside to intervene in case of clinical deterioration per Pediatric Advance Life Support

(PALS) guidelines. Informed consent for surgery must be obtained with the parents or guardian either in person or via telephone.

One common routine elective operation in neonates is gastrostomy tube placement. A gastrostomy tube or "g-tube" is a small feeding tube that is surgically or percutaneously placed in the stomach for feeding or decompression of air or drainage. Surgical placement is either laparoscopic or open and may be done in association with other procedures [29]. Gastrostomy tubes may be needed for preterm neonates with continued inadequate oral feeding once corrected to term if gastrostomy tube feeding is expected to be needed for greater than 4 weeks. Prior to gastrostomy tube placement, the surgeon may request radiographs to evaluate anatomy of the upper gastrointestinal tract. After gastrostomy tube placement, the neonate may have minor pain at the incision site. Intravenous fluids may be required for the first 24 hour to provide parenteral nutrition to allow the site to heal. Generally, the neonate may be restarted on previous feeds at 25% of the total expected volume, and advanced gradually to full enteral feeds via the g-tube within 24–36 hours as tolerated.. A frequent complication of gastrostomy tubes includes dislodgment, usually within the first 2 weeks after its placement [29]. When this occurs, a physician should replace the tube as soon as possible, so the hole in the stomach does not close. A small amount of leaking is normal and may require protective cream application to the skin. A gastrostomy tube may be left in place permanently or temporarily dependent on the neonate's needs [29].

Another common elective surgical procedure includes inguinal hernia repair. An inguinal hernia repair is an internal opening in the inguinal canal through which fluids and/or intestines may pass through [30]. The neonate may have minor pain at the incision site postoperatively that should be controlled with acetaminophen or small doses of morphine. Neonates should be monitored for postoperative respiratory complications such as apnea and oxygen desaturation. Neonates at risk include those with a history of prematurity, especially if still less than 45 weeks corrected gestational age, and neonates with comorbidities including chronic lung disease, history of necrotizing enterocolitis, anemia, low birth weight or former apnea episodes [31, 32]. Healthy, older neonates may generally be repaired as an outpatient [31].

4. Postoperative care of the neonate

Postoperative management should begin with face-to-face communication between the senior clinician caring for the neonate after surgery and the surgeon as well as the anesthesiologist. The neonatologist should be informed of major events that may have occurred during the surgery, the surgery that was performed, the anesthesia the neonate received during the surgery and postoperatively in recovery (especially if paralytic agents were used), as well as the volume and type of fluids or blood products given during the operation.

Temperature homeostasis is important in the postoperative period. Neonates undergoing operative procedures in the operating room are at increased risk of thermal instability. Hypothermia of postoperative neonates leads to an increased risk of adverse respiratory events including increased need for respiratory and cardiac interventions compared to normothermic neonates [33]. Furthermore, hypothermia may cause protein catabolism, hypokalemia and changes in glucose metabolism. Postoperative interventions include applying warm temperature regulating blankets, decreasing skin exposure and warming operative rooms [34].

If the neonate remains intubated postoperatively, obtain a blood gas and chest radiography immediately following return to the ICU to assess oxygenation, ventilation, chest expansion and endotracheal tube position. It is important for clinicians to understand postoperative neonates are prone to apnea and periodic breathing while recovering from anesthesia and in response to pain and pain medications. Neonates are also prone to hypoxemia due to transient decrease in functional residual capacity of the lungs and ventilation/perfusion mismatch. Adequate lung tidal volumes of 6–8 mL/kg expiratory lung volumes should be maintained to prevent atelectasis. Blood gas pH should be maintained at 7.35–7.45 with pCO2 of 40–55 for most neonates. Once the neonate is awake and consistently breathing spontaneously, the clinician should rapidly wean the ventilator and extubate per blood gases if possible. Weaning off mechanical ventilation should be weighed against the need for additional pain control. Surgery should be made aware of neonates requiring nasal continuous positive airway pressure (CPAP) or nasal intermittent mandatory ventilation (IMV) postextubation. Ideally, continuous narcotic infusion for pain control should be at a minimum or discontinued prior to extubation. The clinician should also monitor for the development of pulmonary hypertension by clinical symptoms, pre- and postductal oxygen gradient and confirm by echocardiography [1].

Immediate postoperative labs should include evaluation of hemoglobin/hematocrit. If blood loss is over 15% and not already replaced during the operative period, clinicians should consider replacing with packed red blood cells [35, 36]. Electrolytes should be evaluated in the immediate postoperative period and also monitored every 6 hours for invasive procedures or every 8–12 hours for less intensive procedures for the first 24-hours postoperatively [1].

Surgical neonates may have significant third-space losses depending on the magnitude of the procedure. Phases of fluid resuscitation change with time postoperatively. In the immediate postoperative time period, fluid and blood replacement is often required. Postoperative days 2–4 are often phases of third spacing and vascular leak during which some element of fluid replacement is required in conjunction with diuretics to help mobilize fluids. Avoidance of massive anasarca is important. Abdominal compartment syndrome is especially important to consider in the context of abdominal closures with decreased perfusion and the potential for decreased urine output. Gastroschisis patients are especially prone to large fluid losses. If total parenteral nutrition is not immediately available, D5 lactated ringers should be given. Initial fluids should be given at 150–175 mL/kg/day. Total parenteral nutrition should be optimized to include protein of 3–4 g/kg/day to minimize catabolic state and promote wound healing. Dextrose may need to be adjusted postoperatively due to hyperglycemia secondary to stress and increased fluid administration. Therefore, Accuchecks should be monitored frequently, and glucose infusion rate (GIR) should be adjusted. GIR should be maintained 4–8 μg/kg/min to maintain blood glucose levels of 100–160 mg/dL. Electrolytes should be normalized as much as possible [5]. Consideration of starting enteral nutrition should be discussed when the neonate shows intestinal readiness, presence of bowel sounds and passing gas. Clinicians should monitor for postoperative ileus from the surgery and/or ileus due to pain medications. Antireflux medications should be avoided in the neonate unless for specific surgical cases such as tracheoesophageal fistula where such medications have proven to be necessary. Reflux medications lead to abnormalities of intestinal flora and have been shown to increase neonatal mortality [37].

Special fluid consideration must be made for those neonates with gastroschisis that have undergone repair. Once they are repaired, their fluid losses significantly decrease, and thus, parenteral nutrition must be adjusted shortly after surgical closure. Total fluid administration should be decreased to approximately 140–150 mL/kg/day [38], based on the assessment of the neonate's fluid losses. Clinicians should be cautious of fluid volumes as overhydration may lengthen hospital stay and delay enteral feeding [38].

Hypotension secondary to hypovolemia may be treated with 10–20 mL/kg boluses of normal saline or if hypotension is persistent and severe, the clinician should consider fresh frozen plasma. If anemic, packed red blood cells may be used. Albumin should rarely be used and only with great caution as it may worsen third-space fluid losses in neonates. Low albumin is often partially dilutional and when not exacerbated by dilutional effects, is best addressed through maximizing protein delivery through nutrition. Replacement of any gastric output should be considered with 0.45 normal saline with 10 mEq of potassium chloride per liter. If output is large, consider replacing more frequently (i.e., every 4 hours to run over 4 hours versus once a shift over 1 hour if lower output). Replacement of gastric fluid is important to maintain fluid balance but must be balanced with urine output and overall body edema. Vasopressor therapy may be considered for the critically ill postoperative neonate if fluid replacement is already optimized and neonate remains hypotensive with signs of decreased end-organ perfusion. Steroid therapy to aid adrenal stress response may also improve hemodynamic stability; however, it should be used cautiously as steroids may decrease immune response if there is concern for infection.

Fluid status must be monitored closely, and urine output should be maintained at a minimum of 1 mL/kg/hour. The clinician must balance the neonate's overall fluid status as measured by weight, urine output, body wall edema, blood pressure, heart rate and overall clinical status. Edematous neonates may still have low intravascular volumes, and thus, diuretics would possibly exacerbate hypotension.

Blood pressure should be monitored closely, at least hourly if there is no arterial line access. Hypotension in the postoperative period is considered a sign of hypovolemia until proven otherwise. Skin perfusion should be monitored which can be done by NIRS or perfusion index of pulse oximetry monitoring. All tubes and drains should be monitored closely postoperatively for patency, function and how secure they are attached to the patient. Output of sumps, chest tubes, wound drains and Foley catheters should be followed. Pending resolution of ileus and improvement in outputs each should be removed at the earliest time point to prevent infection with persistent foreign bodies.

Prevention of infection is important. White blood cell count, C-reactive protein trend and bandemia should be monitored and blood cultures obtained if concern for infection rises [1]. Be especially cautious of hygienic precautions when handling tubes, drains and any wound dressing changes. The need for postoperative antibiotic coverage should be discussed between the neonatal clinician and surgeon.

5. Pain management, sedation and paralysis review

Pain control should be titrated based on the type of surgery. More invasive surgeries will likely require immediate postoperative pain management including a narcotic drip for the first 24 – 48 hours [39]. Consider morphine 20-50 micrograms/kg/hour or Fentanyl 3 micrograms/kg/hour with as needed (PRN) dosing for breakthrough pain. Pain management should be transitioned to PRN dosing when able. Titration of pain medication should be assessed through reliable and accurate neonatal pain assessment scoring tools such as the "Neonatal Pain, Agitation and Sedation Scale" (N-PASS) [40] or "Crying, Requires increased oxygen administration, Increased vital signs, Expression and Sleeplessness" (CRIES) [41]. A combination of behavioral observations such as facial expression, body posture and tone and physiologic symptoms such as heart rate, blood pressure and oxygen saturation should be taken into consideration by the neonatal pain score used [22].

Nonnarcotic pain management methods should be used such as Sweet-Ease and intravenous Tylenol 20 mg/kg/dose every 6 hours for a 24-48 hour period, unless contraindicated or if there is concern for liver dysfunction. The neonate should be monitored closely for urinary retention if Foley catheter is not in place. The stomach should be decompressed. Nonpharmacological pain management includes protective neonatal positioning if possible with the neonate supported in the flex position. Environmental stimulation should be minimized with decreased lighting, noise and touch.

Use of chemical paralytic agents postoperatively should only be used in cases where there is concern for wound dehiscence, large irreducible gastroschisis or patient instability. Paralytics should be used for shortest time possible, as the use will increase the likelihood of third-spacing fluids, urinary retention and anasarca [39].

6. Follow-up of the surgical neonate

The care of a neonate following discharge from the ICU is one that requires a multidisciplinary approach. The patient's pediatrician, neonatologist in the High Risk Follow Clinic (when appropriate), various therapists and the primary surgeon will need to see the neonate after discharge [42]. Follow-up visits include neurodevelopment assessment scales using Bayley III and WPPSI-II scores. While there are certain risk factors innate to sick neonates that make them prone to developmental delay such as prematurity and/or congenital defects, there are data to suggest that neonates who require surgical intervention experience initial developmental delays as compared with their healthy counterparts [43]. While there is ample evidence of suboptimal developmental outcomes in neonates requiring cardiac surgery, the data for those undergoing repair of conditions such as gastroschisis suggest that outcomes are similar to those of their healthy cohorts [44]. Those neonates who have had significant surgical intervention and those with severe outcomes such as short gut syndrome require a lifelong close follow-up with the surgical team.

http://dx.doi.org/10.5772/67174

Author details

Shelly Haug*, Sara Farooqi, Anamika Banerji and Andrew Hopper

*Address all correspondence to: shaug@llu.edu

Loma Linda University Children's Hospital, Loma Linda, CA, USA

References

[1] Philadelphia TCH of Perioperative Care Newborns/Infants—Clinical Pathway: ICU and Inpatient. http://www.chop.edu/clinical-pathway/perioperative-care-newborns-infants-clinical-pathway. Published August 12, 2014. Accessed October 23, 2016.

[2] Rowe MI, Rowe SA. The last fifty years of neonatal surgical management. *Am J Surg*. 2000;180(5):345–352.

[3] Percutaneous Placement of Central Venous Catheters. University of Iowa Children's Hospital. https://uichildrens.org/health-library/percutaneous-placement-central-venous-catheters. Published September 12, 2012. Accessed November 27, 2016.

[4] American Society of Anesthesiologists Committee. Practice guidelines for preoperative fasting and the use of pharmacologic agents to reduce the risk of pulmonary aspiration: application to healthy patients undergoing elective procedures: an updated report by the American Society of Anesthesiologists Committee on Standards and Practice Parameters. *Anesthesiology*. 2011;114(3):495–511. doi:10.1097/ALN.0b013e3181fcbfd9

[5] Dell KM. Fluid, Electrolytes, and Acid-Base Homeostasis. In R. J. Martin, A. A. Fanaroff, & M. C. Walsh (Authors), Fanaroff and Martin's neonatal-perinatal medicine: diseases of the fetus and infant. Philadelphia, PA: Elsevier/Saunders. 2015;613–627.

[6] Bell EF, Warburton D, Stonestreet BS, Oh W. High-volume fluid intake predisposes premature infants to necrotising enterocolitis. *Lancet Lond Engl*. 1979;2(8133):90.

[7] Bell EF, Warburton D, Stonestreet BS, Oh W. Effect of fluid administration on the development of symptomatic patent ductus arteriosus and congestive heart failure in premature infants. *N Engl J Med*. 1980;302(11):598–604. doi:10.1056/NEJM198003133021103

[8] Marshall DD, Kotelchuck M, Young TE, et al. Risk factors for chronic lung disease in the surfactant era: a North Carolina population-based study of very low birth weight infants. *Pediatrics*. 1999;104(6):1345–1350. doi:10.1542/peds.104.6.1345

[9] Piasek CZ, Van Bel F, Sola A. Perfusion index in newborn infants: a noninvasive tool for neonatal monitoring. *Acta Paediatr Oslo Nor 1992*. 2014;103(5):468–473. doi:10.1111/apa.12574

[10] Terek D, Altun Koroglu O, Ulger Z, Yalaz M, Kultursay N. The serial changes of perfusion index in preterm infants with patent ductus arteriosus: is perfusion index clinically significant? *Minerva Pediatr*. 2016;68(4):250–255.

[11] Koch HW, Hansen TG. Perioperative use of cerebral and renal near-infrared spectroscopy in neonates: a 24-h observational study. *Pediatr Anesth*. 2016;26(2):190–198. doi:10.1111/pan.12831

[12] Alderliesten T, Dix L, Baerts W, et al. Reference values of regional cerebral oxygen saturation during the first 3 days of life in preterm neonates. *Pediatr Res*. 2016;79(1–1):55–64. doi:10.1038/pr.2015.186

[13] Chock V. NIRS Educational Module. November 2016. http://neonatology.stanford.edu/content/dam/sm/neonatology/documents/NIRS%20Educational%20Module.pdf.

[14] McNeill S, Gatenby JC, McElroy S, Engelhardt B. Normal cerebral, renal and abdominal regional oxygen saturations using near-infrared spectroscopy in preterm infants. *J Perinatol*. 2011;31(1):51–57. doi:10.1038/jp.2010.71

[15] Wilson RD, Johnson MP. Congenital abdominal wall defects: an update. *Fetal Diagn Ther*. 2004;19(5):385–398. doi:10.1159/000078990

[16] Lund CH, Bauer K, Berrios M. Gastroschisis: incidence, complications, and clinical management in the neonatal intensive care unit. *J Perinat Neonatal Nurs*. 2007;21(1):63–68.

[17] O'Connell RV, Dotters-Katz SK, Kuller JA, Strauss RA. Gastroschisis: a review of management and outcomes. *Obstet Gynecol Surv*. 2016;71(9):537–544. doi:10.1097/OGX.0000000000000344

[18] Bonasso PC, Lucke-Wold B, Hobbs GR, Vaughan RA, Shorter NA, Nakayama DK. Excessive postoperative fluid administration in infants with gastroschisis. *Am Surg*. 2016;82(8):704–706.

[19] McNair C, Hawes J, Urquhart H. Caring for the newborn with an omphalocele. *Neonatal Netw NN*. 2006;25(5):319–327. doi:10.1891/0730-0832.25.5.319

[20] Philippart AI, Canty TG, Filler RM. Acute fluid volume requirements in infants with anterior abdominal wall defects. *J Pediatr Surg*. 1972;7(5):553–558. doi:10.1016/0022-3468(72)90212-6

[21] Baerg JE, Thorpe DL, Sharp NE, et al. Pulmonary hypertension predicts mortality in infants with omphalocele. *J Neonatal-Perinat Med*. 2015;8(4):333–338. doi:10.3233/NPM-15915011

[22] Bhalla T, Shepherd E, Tobias JD. Neonatal pain management. *Saudi J Anaesth*. 2014;8(Suppl 1):S89–S97. doi:10.4103/1658-354X.144085

[23] Spatz DL, Schmidt KJ. Breastfeeding success in infants with giant omphalocele. *Adv Neonatal Care Off J Natl Assoc Neonatal Nurses*. 2012;12(6):329–335. doi:10.1097/ANC.0b013e31826150c5

[24] Haug S, St Peter S, Ramlogan S, et al. The impact of breast milk, respiratory insufficiency and GERD on enteral feeding in infants with omphalocele. *J Pediatr Gastroenterol Nutr*. November 2016. doi:10.1097/MPG.0000000000001463

[25] Kimura K, Loening-Baucke V. Bilious vomiting in the newborn: rapid diagnosis of intestinal obstruction. *Am Fam Physician*. 2000;61(9):2791–2798.

[26] Neu J, Walker WA. Necrotizing Enterocolitis. *N Engl J Med*. 2011;364(3):255–264. doi:10.1056/NEJMra1005408

[27] Fitzgibbons SC, Ching Y, Yu D, et al. Mortality of necrotizing enterocolitis expressed by birth weight categories. *J Pediatr Surg*. 2009;44(6):1072–1076. doi:10.1016/j.jpedsurg.2009.02.013

[28] Neu J. Necrotizing enterocolitis: the search for a unifying pathogenic theory leading to prevention. *Pediatr Clin North Am*. 1996;43(2):409–432.

[29] Gastrostomy (G-Tube) Surgery | Children's Hospital Pittsburgh. Children's Hospital of Pittsburgh. http://www.chp.edu/our-services/transplant/intestine/education/patient-procedures/gastrostomy. Accessed November 23, 2016.

[30] Inguinal Hernia Repair Surgery | Children's Hospital Pittsburgh. Children's Hospital of Pittsburgh. http://www.chp.edu/our-services/urology/patient-procedures/hernia. Accessed November 23, 2016.

[31] Özdemir T, Arıkan A. Postoperative apnea after inguinal hernia repair in formerly premature infants: impacts of gestational age, postconceptional age and comorbidities. *Pediatr Surg Int*. 2013;29(8):801–804. doi:10.1007/s00383-013-3330-8

[32] Murphy JJ, Swanson T, Ansermino M, Milner R. The frequency of apneas in premature infants after inguinal hernia repair: do they need overnight monitoring in the intensive care unit? *J Pediatr Surg*. 2008;43(5):865–868. doi:10.1016/j.jpedsurg.2007.12.028

[33] Morehouse D, Williams L, Lloyd C, et al. Perioperative hypothermia in NICU infants: its occurrence and impact on infant outcomes. *Adv Neonatal Care Off J Natl Assoc Neonatal Nurses*. 2014;14(3):154–164. doi:10.1097/ANC.0000000000000045

[34] Dennison D. Thermal regulation of patients during the perioperative period. *AORN J*. 1995;61(5):827–828, 831–832.

[35] Fasano R, Luban NLC. Blood component therapy. *Pediatr Clin North Am*. 2008;55(2):421–445. doi:10.1016/j.pcl.2008.01.006

[36] Roseff SD, Luban NLC, Manno CS. Guidelines for assessing appropriateness of pediatric transfusion. *Transfusion (Paris)*. 2002;42(11):1398–1413. doi:10.1046/j.1537-2995.2002.00208.x

[37] Terrin G, Passariello A, Curtis MD, et al. Ranitidine is associated with infections, necrotizing enterocolitis, and fatal outcome in newborns. *Pediatrics*. 2012;129(1):e40–e45. doi:10.1542/peds.2011-0796

[38] Waldhausen JHT. Surgical management of gastroschisis. *NeoReviews*. 2005;6(11):e500–e507. doi:10.1542/neo.6-11-e500

[39] Committee on Fetus And Newborn and Section on Anesthesiology and Pain Medicine. Prevention and management of procedural pain in the neonate: an update. *Pediatrics*. 2016;137(2):e20154271. doi:10.1542/peds.2015-4271

[40] Hillman BA, Tabrizi MN, Gauda EB, Carson KA, Aucott SW. The Neonatal Pain, Agitation and Sedation Scale and the bedside nurse's assessment of neonates. *J Perinatol Off J Calif Perinat Assoc*. 2015;35(2):128–131. doi:10.1038/jp.2014.154

[41] Krechel SW, Bildner J. CRIES: a new neonatal postoperative pain measurement score. Initial testing of validity and reliability. *Paediatr Anaesth*. 1995;5(1):53–61.

[42] Panel SA. Referral to pediatric surgical specialists. *Pediatrics*. 2014;133(2):350–356. doi:10.1542/peds.2013-3820

[43] Ludman L, Spitz L, Landsdown R. Developmental progress of newborns undergoing neonatal surgery. *J Pediatr Surg*. 1990;25(5):469–471. doi:10.1016/0022-3468(90)90552-K

[44] Harris EL, Hart SJ, Minutillo C, et al. The long-term neurodevelopmental and psychological outcomes of gastroschisis: A cohort study. *J Pediatr Surg*. 2016;51(4):549–553. doi:10.1016/j.jpedsurg.2015.08.062

[45] Fanaroff AA, Martin FJ (eds). Neonatal and Perinatal Medicine: Diseases of the Fetus and Newborn (10th edition). St. Louis: Mosby; 1997, p 672.

Section 2

Anesthetic Management for Neonates and Children

Chapter 2

Anesthetic Management of the Newborn Surgical Patient

Marissa Vadi, Chelan Nour, Patrick Leiter and Harmony Carter

Additional information is available at the end of the chapter

http://dx.doi.org/10.5772/66932

Abstract

Providing anesthesia for the newborn requires many considerations beyond what is needed for the older child or adult. This chapter discusses pertinent anesthetic considerations in the care of surgical neonates including preoperative evaluation, intraoperative management and pain management techniques.

Keywords: neonatal anesthesia, anesthetic agents, pain management

1. Introduction

Advances in pediatric anesthesiology have contributed to improved outcomes and survival in newborns requiring surgical intervention. Newborn physiology is characterized by a high metabolic rate, limited cardiopulmonary reserve, and decreased renal function. Multisystem organ immaturity underlies the differences in physiologic response to anesthetics in the neonate when compared to the older child or adult. This chapter discusses physiologic considerations, preoperative evaluation and preparation, intraoperative anesthetic management, and pain management techniques unique to the newborn surgical patient.

2. Physiologic considerations

2.1. Cardiovascular

Fetal cardiac circulation is characterized by two right-to-left shunts: one through the foramen ovale and one through the ductus arteriosus. With the infant's first breaths, the lungs expand, alveolar fluid is cleared, pulmonary vascular resistance markedly decreases, and left atrial pressure increases [1]. These physiologic changes promote functional closure of the fetal cardiac shunts and mark the beginning of the transition from fetal to newborn circulation.

Anatomic closure of the foramen ovale typically occurs within the first year of life, though some studies indicate over one quarter of foramen ovale remain echocardiography probe patent into adulthood [2]. Functional closure of the ductus arteriosus is achieved between 10 and 15 hours of life, and anatomical closure is usually completed by 2 months of age [3]. Neonatal circulation may revert to fetal circulation if the physiological parameters responsible for cardiac shunt closure are not maintained. As such, it is important to avoid factors that increase pulmonary vascular resistance (physiologic stress, hypoxia, hypercarbia, acidosis, and hypothermia) in newborns. Hypervolemia may also promote reopening of the ductus arteriosus and should be avoided.

Maintenance of heart rate is essential in the neonatal period. Cardiac output is dependent on heart rate, as stroke volume is fixed due to decreased compliance of the immature ventricle [4]. Thus, while maintaining preload is important during anesthetic management, increasing preload provides minimal benefit for improving cardiac output. The sympathetic nervous system is also immature in newborns. Bradycardia may occur after stimulating procedures such as laryngoscopy, oropharyngeal suctioning, or gastric tube placement rather than the expected tachycardia seen in patients with mature sympathetic nervous systems. Treatment with anticholinergics may be required.

2.2. Pulmonary

Development of the respiratory system begins during fetal organogenesis and continues throughout childhood. Alveolarization starts at 28 weeks of gestational age, and by 40 weeks, alveoli are present at 20–50% of adult values. Type 2 pneumocytes, the main producers of surfactant, appear at approximately 24 weeks of gestational age but are not fully functional until 34–36 weeks of gestational age [5].

Neonates are an increased risk for respiratory fatigue. High chest wall compliance may cause a paradoxical breathing pattern when large breaths are taken [5]. Newborns have a reduced number of fatigue-resistant high-oxidative diaphragmatic muscle fibers; mature levels are not reached until 8 months of age [6]. Neonatal oxygen requirements are 2–3 times the adult requirement, ranging from 6 to 9 mL/kg/min. Increased oxygen demand is met by increased respiratory rate, as there is a minimal inspiratory reserve to increase tidal volume [7].

Neonatal respiratory drive is determined by pO_2 via peripheral chemoreceptors in the carotid bodies and by pCO_2 influencing central chemoreceptors in the medulla. Respiratory drive is primarily affected by hypoxia, as opposed to hypercarbia in adults. Administration of high oxygen concentrations may depress respiratory drive in the newborn [8].

2.3. Renal

The kidneys are fully developed anatomically by 34–36 weeks of gestational age but continue to develop functionally after birth. The glomerular filtration rate (GFR) is initially decreased

http://dx.doi.org/10.5772/66932

in the neonate due to low systemic arterial pressure and high renal vascular resistance but increases during the first several weeks of extrauterine life [9]. As a result of this initial low GFR, there is a decreased ability of the kidneys to maintain electrolyte balance or clear drugs and excess fluids.

2.4. Neurologic risk

The neurologic system is anatomically complete at term, though synaptogenesis and nerve myelination continue throughout childhood. Data from animal studies, as well as retrospective human studies, have raised concern that exposure to anesthetic agents could be detrimental to cognitive development in young children due to effects either on synaptogenesis or apoptosis of the developing brain [10]. The stage of brain development at the time of exposure and the degree of anesthetic exposure, in terms of both exposure frequency and cumulative anesthetic dose, may affect the risk of neurotoxicity.

The SmartTots program, a partnership between the United States Food and Drug Administration and the International Anesthesia Research Society, was established in 2009 to address the growing concern regarding potential adverse consequences of general anesthesia in young children. Two consensus statements, published in 2012 and 2015, counsel that the effect of exposure to anesthetic drugs in young children is unknown. Some, but not all, studies to date have suggested that problems similar to those seen in animals could also occur in infants and toddlers. The benefits of elective procedures must be weighed against the risks associated with anesthesia and surgery [11].

3. Preoperative evaluation and preparation

3.1. History and physical examination

A thorough preanesthetic history and physical examination must be performed with the goals of identifying potential anesthetic complications due to coexisting disease, determining whether further diagnostic studies are required prior to surgery and anticipating postoperative concerns including pain management and level of cardiorespiratory monitoring required.

Factors that should be addressed in the preanesthetic history are outlined in **Table 1**. A review of all organ systems, including identification of genetic syndromes and associated anomalies, should be completed. Examination of previous anesthetic and surgical records may reveal difficulties with airway management, venous access, or anesthetic emergence and assist in planning future anesthetic management.

Physical examination should assess for evidence of coexisting diseases (e.g., craniofacial abnormalities, congenital heart disease, chronic lung disease). Hydration status may be determined by evaluating skin turgor, mucous membranes, fontanelle fullness, and urine output. Existing intravenous catheters should be examined for patency and hypovolemia treated prior to anesthetic induction. Laboratory studies must be reviewed and significant electrolyte abnormalities and/or anemia corrected preoperatively.

The American Society of Anesthesiologists (ASA) physical status classification system is used as a uniform system for describing the degree of patient morbidity prior to an anesthetic (**Table 2**) [12]. The grading system is not intended for use as a measure to predict operative risk.

Factor	Specific concerns
Maternal history during pregnancy	Rh-ABO compatibility
	Diabetes
	Toxemia
	Infection
	Drug or alcohol abuse
Gestational age and weight	Extreme prematurity and/or extremely low birth weight
Significant birth events	Apgar scores
	Neonatal asphyxia
	Meconium aspiration
Perinatal course	Apneas
	Supplemental oxygen requirement
	Need for ventilator support
Medications and medication allergies	Type and severity of adverse medication reaction

Table 1. Factors to address in the preanesthetic history.

Physical score classification*	Definition
ASA I	A normal healthy patient
ASA II	A patient with mild systemic disease
ASA III	A patient with severe systemic disease
ASA IV	A patient with severe systemic disease that is a constant threat to life
ASA V	A moribund patient who is not expected to survive without the operation
ASA VI	A declared brain-dead patient whose organs are being removed for donor purposes

*Emergency cases are designated by the addition of "E" to the classification number.

Table 2. American Society of Anesthesiologists physical status classification system.

3.2. Fasting

Infants are required to fast before procedures requiring sedation and anesthesia in order to minimize the risk of pulmonary aspiration of gastric contents [13]. Fasting times are based on pediatric gastric emptying studies. **Table 3** provides a summary of fasting recommendations by the ASA [14]. Prolonged fasting may lead to hypovolemia and hypoglycemia in infants; glucose-containing intravenous maintenance fluids should be administered prior to the induction of anesthesia.

The majority of pediatric aspiration events occur during anesthetic induction [15]. Risk factors for aspiration in the perianesthetic period include neurologic abnormality, emergency surgery, intestinal obstruction or increased abdominal pressure, light anesthesia, and the skill of the anesthesia provider [16, 17]. Infants and young children are particularly prone to regurgitation and aspiration for a variety of reasons including air swallowing while crying and decreased lower esophageal sphincter incompetence. In one study, almost all cases of pulmonary aspiration occurred in children who gagged or coughed during airway management, either because neuromuscular blockade was not administered or airway manipulation occurred before the child was completely paralyzed [15]. Mortality due to pulmonary aspiration is low, with an estimated incidence between zero and 1:50,000 [15, 16, 18].

Ingested material	Minimum fasting period (hours)
Clear liquids	2
Breast milk	4
Infant formula	6
Nonhuman milk	6
Light meal	6

Table 3. American Society of Anesthesiologists fasting recommendations.

3.3. Postoperative apnea in former premature infants

Postoperative apnea is defined as cessation of breathing or no detectable airflow for 15 seconds or longer, or less than 15 seconds with bradycardia. It has been observed in former premature infants after exposure to all forms of anesthetics (intravenous agents, inhalational agents, and regional anesthesia) [19–21]. The incidence of postoperative apnea varies inversely with gestational age at birth and post-conceptual age at the time of surgery. Apnea risk is greater than 1% until 54 weeks of post-conceptual age or 56 weeks of post-conceptual age in infants with a gestational age of 32 or 35 weeks, respectively [22].

Former preterm infants who are less than 60 weeks of post-conceptual age at the time of surgery should be monitored until free of apnea for at least 12 hours. A monitored bed should be arranged for the postoperative period, and family members should be educated regarding the risk of perianesthesia apnea. Children receiving theophylline or caffeine preoperatively should have these medications continued postoperatively [23]. Caffeine administration does not negate the need for postoperative respiratory monitoring. Factors such as anemia, hypothermia, hypoglycemia, hypocalcemia, acidosis, and hypoxemia may increase the risk of apnea and should be avoided.

4. Intraoperative management

4.1. Monitoring and intravenous access

The ASA's Standards for Basic Anesthetic Monitoring mandates continual evaluation of oxygenation, ventilation, circulation, and temperature during all anesthetics [24]. Placement of both a pre-ductal oxygen saturation monitor on the right upper extremity and a post-ductal oxygen saturation monitor on a lower extremity should be considered in neonates as a means to detect right-to-left shunting across the ductus arteriosus [25]. A nerve stimulator may be used if neuromuscular blocking agents are administered, though the train-of-four response is often diminished in infants less than 2 months old. It is imperative that the operating room be kept warm. Neonates, especially premature infants, are at high risk for heat loss due to an increased surface area to volume ratio when compared to older children and adults [26, 27]. The need for invasive monitoring, including arterial and central venous catheter placement, is determined by the baseline medical condition of the patient and the extensiveness of the planned surgery. Arterial catheters allow for continuous monitoring of heart rate and blood pressure, as well as arterial blood gas sampling [28]. Central venous catheters are utilized when large intravenous access is necessary, central venous pressure monitoring is required, or in hemodynamically unstable conditions likely to require continuous vasopressor infusions. The benefits of placement must always be weighed against the risks associated with use, such as catheter-associated bloodstream infection [29]. A urinary catheter should be considered in surgical cases of prolonged duration or when significant blood loss is expected.

4.2. Anesthetic agents

Most infants arriving as outpatients for surgery may undergo mask induction of anesthesia with inhaled anesthetic agents. Those patients presenting from inpatient hospital wards or the neonatal intensive care unit (NICU) with intravenous access in situ may undergo intravenous induction of general anesthesia [27].

4.2.1. Inhaled anesthetic agents

Inhaled halogenated anesthetics (most commonly sevoflurane, isoflurane, and desflurane) are used for both induction and maintenance of general anesthesia. The minimum alveolar concentration (MAC) is the end-tidal concentration of inhaled anesthetic agent at which 50% of patients do not move in response to a noxious stimulus. MAC values are used to compare the relative potencies of anesthetic agents and vary with age for each particular agent (**Table 4**) [30–32]. Of note, MAC values may differ for preterm neonates depending upon the inhalational agent used and the gestational age of the infant.

Sevoflurane is the halogenated agent most commonly chosen for mask induction of anesthesia; its use is associated with a reduced incidence of breath holding, coughing, laryngospasm, and oxygen desaturation when compared with other inhaled anesthetics [30]. Nitrous oxide, a nonhalogenated agent, may be used in conjunction with halogenated

Characteristic	Sevoflurane	Desflurane	Isoflurane	Nitrous oxide
MAC adult	2.05%	7.0%	1.2%	104%
MAC neonate (full term)	3.2%	9.2%	1.6%	–

Table 4. Minimum alveolar concentration (MAC) values for modern inhalational anesthetics.

inhaled anesthetics to speed inhalational induction ("second-gas effect") or reduce halogenated agent doses during the maintenance phase of anesthesia. Nitrous oxide must be used with caution as it may rapidly diffuse into and expand gas-filled body cavities. Its use should be avoided in laparoscopic surgery and is contraindicated in patients with a pneumothorax [33].

4.2.2. *Intravenous anesthetic agents*

Similar to inhaled halogenated anesthetics, intravenous anesthetic agents may be utilized for both induction and maintenance of anesthesia. Agent choice is commonly based upon the following drug properties: speed of onset, duration of action, cardiovascular stability, and side-effect profile [34].

Propofol is an intravenous agent with sedative-hypnotic properties resulting from gamma-aminobutyric acid (GABA)-mediated inhibitory neurotransmission. Systolic blood pressure falls approximately 15% after propofol administration due to decreases in preload, cardiac contractility, and systemic vascular resistance. Propofol is a potent respiratory depressant, and apnea may occur transiently after bolus administration. Pain on injection may be attenuated with intravenous lidocaine administration.

Ketamine is a phencyclidine derivative that antagonizes N-methyl-D-aspartate (NMDA) receptors. This results in a "dissociative"-type anesthesia and a potential for disturbing dreams or delirium. Ketamine possesses excellent amnestic, analgesic, and bronchodilation properties. Administration is associated with favorable hemodynamic parameters except in catecholamine-depleted patients. The use is limited in patients with a history of seizure disorder and in those in whom increases in intracranial and/or intraocular pressures would be detrimental. Nystagmus, myoclonus, and copious oral secretions are frequent side effects of ketamine use.

Etomidate depresses the reticular activating system and mimics the inhibitory effects of GABA. It possesses minimal effects on the hemodynamic system but can decrease ventilatory drive. Induction doses are known to transiently inhibit enzymes involved in cortisol and aldosterone synthesis with the potential for adrenocortical suppression.

Thiopental is a barbiturate that acts by prolonging the duration of GABA-mediated chloride channel opening. Administration can cause cardiovascular depression that is accentuated in the hypovolemic patient. Compared to other induction agents, acute tolerance to thiopental may develop, and prolonged sedation can be noted after induction doses [35].

4.2.3. Neuromuscular blocking agents

Neuromuscular blocking drugs allow for patient immobility, smooth endotracheal intubation, increased tolerance of mechanical ventilation, and optimal surgical relaxation. They are classified into two groups, depolarizing and non-depolarizing agents, based on activity at the neuromuscular junction [36]. The choice of drug depends on the desired speed of onset, duration of action, route of elimination, and side-effect profile.

Succinylcholine is the only depolarizing agent currently available for clinical use. An increased dose of succinylcholine is necessary in infants due to relative effect resistance at the neuromuscular junction and the larger volume of distribution in the neonate. Succinylcholine is metabolized by circulating pseudocholinesterase. It has a very rapid onset (60 seconds) and short duration of action (5 minutes). Succinylcholine carries an FDA "black box warning" against routine use in children due to risk of hyperkalemic cardiac arrest in patients with undiagnosed neuromuscular disorders [37]. Thus, it is recommended that the use of succinylcholine in children be reserved for emergency intubation or instances where immediate securing of the airway is necessary (e.g., laryngospasm, difficulty airway, full stomach) [38].

Non-depolarizing neuromuscular blocking agents are divided into intermediate (atracurium, cisatracurium, rocuronium, and vecuronium) and long-acting (pancuronium) varieties [26]. Neuromuscular blocking drugs are responsible for over 35% of anesthetic-related hypersensitivity reactions and should be considered as potential causes if anaphylaxis is suspected in the perianesthetic period. The effects of non-depolarizing muscle relaxants may be antagonized by an anticholinesterase (neostigmine or edrophonium) administered in conjunction with an anticholinergic agent (glycopyrrolate or atropine) to minimize parasympathetic side effects. Successful reversal of neuromuscular blockade in infants is demonstrated by adequate return of strong hip and/or arm flexion, abdominal muscle contraction, and return of the train-of-four twitch response to four equal twitches.

Historically, neuromuscular blocking drugs could only be reversed after adequate time had elapsed to demonstrate some natural return of neuromuscular function. Sugammadex, a cyclodextrin oligosaccharide, is a new reversal agent that inactivates steroidal neuromuscular blocking agents such as vecuronium and rocuronium via direct encapsulation. This mechanism allows for rapid and complete reversal of neuromuscular blockade within minutes of administration of a neuromuscular blocking agent. Studies examining sugammadex use in children aged 2–18 years suggest no evidence of higher incidence of adverse effects with sugammadex compared to that with neostigmine or placebo [39]. Data regarding the safety of sugammadex in infants are currently limited.

4.3. Fluid and blood product management

Calculating total intraoperative fluid requirements necessitates considering fluid type, maintenance fluid requirements, evaporative fluid losses, and replacement of intraoperative blood loss.

4.3.1. Glucose requirements

Healthy infants and children can remain euglycemic for up to 17 hours despite fasting. Infants receiving total parenteral nutrition or 10% dextrose in water (D10W) preoperatively require continued glucose replacement intraoperatively [27, 40]. Glucose levels naturally increase intraoperatively secondary to decreased insulin sensitivity from release of surgery-related stress hormones.

4.3.2. Maintenance fluid requirements

Maintenance fluid requirements are determined by accounting for water losses from the renal, pulmonary, and gastrointestinal systems in addition to calculating baseline body weight and calorie usage [40]. While a variety of formulas exist to determine the maintenance fluid requirements of an infant or child, the simplest is the "4-2-1" rule shown in **Table 5** [40, 41].

D5 0.25% normal saline (NS) and D5 0.45% NS are commonly chosen maintenance fluids for children, as they closely accomplish the goal of delivering 3 mEq of sodium, 2 mEq of potassium, 2 mEq of chloride, and 5 g of glucose for every 100 mL of water administered. *Nil per os* (NPO) fluid deficit is calculated by multiplying the hourly maintenance fluid requirement by the number of hours the patient has been NPO. The NPO deficit is typically replaced intraoperatively as follows: half the total volume deficit is administered in the first hour, one quarter in the second hour, and the remaining quarter in the third hour.

Intraoperative evaporative fluid losses may be replenished with isotonic crystalloid or colloid fluids according to the following formula based on the invasiveness of surgery: superficial 1–2 mL/kg/h, moderate/intrathoracic 4–7 mL/kg/h, open intra-abdominal 6–10 mL/kg/h, and neonates with necrotizing enterocolitis >50 mL/kg/h. Current data are limited but do not support specific benefits of human albumin usage over other colloids or crystalloids in neonates [42, 43]. Favored colloid usage is institutional and region specific; many centers in the United States utilize albumin, while institutions in other nations favor hydroxyethyl starches or gelatins [44].

Weight	Hourly	Day
<10 kg	4 mL/kg	100 mL/kg
10–20 kg	40 mL + 2 mL/kg for every kg >10 kg	1 L + 50 mL/kg for every kg >10 kg
>20 kg	60 mL + 1 mL/kg for every kg >20 kg	1.5 L + 20 mL/kg for every kg >20 kg

Table 5. Maintenance fluid requirements by weight.

4.3.3. Blood products

Estimated blood volume is calculated based on the age and weight of the patient (**Table 6**) [45]. Prior to surgery, one may calculate the maximum allowable blood loss (MABL) that would necessitate blood transfusion using the following equation:

$$\text{MABL} = EBV \times \frac{(Hct\,\text{current} - Hct\,\text{min})}{(Hct\,\text{current})} \tag{1}$$

where *Hct current* is the current hematocrit and *Hct min* is the minimum acceptable hematocrit.

Age	Estimated blood volume (mL/kg)
Premature infant (<37 weeks of gestational age)	100
Term infant	90
Toddler	80
School-aged child	75
Adult	65–70

Table 6. Calculating estimated blood volume.

Recommended doses for replacement of blood products are outlined in **Table 7** [46].

Packed red blood cells (PRBCs) have a hematocrit of approximately 55–70%. Fresh frozen plasma (FFP) administration is indicated when there is laboratory evidence of coagulopathy or significant blood loss approaching one blood volume [47]. Intraoperative platelet transfusion is more likely to be necessary with preoperative platelet counts <150,000 per mm^3 or after the loss of two to three blood volumes [41, 48]. Massive blood loss has historically been replaced in a 1:1:1 fashion with PRBCs, FFP, and platelets. Currently, it is recommended that FFP administration begins after one blood volume has been lost or at the first sign of clinical coagulopathy [49]. It is imperative for the surgeon and the anesthesiologist to maintain excellent communication regarding expectations for blood loss and proper preparation of the patient including any necessary laboratory screening tests for blood typing, antibodies, and cross matching.

Product	Dose	Expected increase
Packed red blood cells	10–15 mL/kg	Hemoglobin 2–3 g/dL
Fresh frozen plasma	10–15 mL/kg	Factors 15–25%
Platelets	5–10 mL/kg	Platelets 50–100,000/mm^3
Cryoprecipitate	1–2 units/kg	Fibrinogen 60–100 mg/dL

Table 7. Recommended doses for replacement of blood products.

5. Neonatal pain management

Pain has been defined as "an unpleasant sensory and emotional experience associated with actual or potential tissue damage, or described in terms of such damage" [50]. Accurately defining and quantifying pain in the neonate has challenged the medical community for decades. Neonatal pain pathways are immature and poorly understood; over 40 different pain scales have been developed to assess pain in the term and preterm neonate. Because neonates and infants cannot verbally communicate pain, regrettably their pain may go unrecognized and undertreated.

Historically, it was believed that neonates did not have the same pain perception as older infants and adults. Opioids were known to cause respiratory depression and were considered harmful; thus, postoperative analgesia with opioids was discouraged. This remained the predominant view until as late as in 1987, when research by Anand and colleagues challenged this long-standing tradition by demonstrating that unattenuated noxious or painful stimuli during neonatal cardiac surgery caused a deleterious stress response and increased morbidity. Anand published two landmark papers presenting scientific evidence that neonates experience pain and the medical necessity for treating such pain. Change in practice soon followed, accompanied by a rapid expansion of literature in this area [51–53].

Neonates in the intensive care unit are estimated to undergo as many as 14 invasive procedures associated with pain each day, with analgesia inconsistently provided for many of these procedures (**Table 8**) [54]. This is concerning as research has correlated undertreated pain in the neonatal period with long-term detrimental effects, including behavioral disorders and altered sensitivity to pain later in life [55–59].

5.1. Pain assessment

An ongoing challenge involves appropriately assessing and effectively treating pain in the neonate. The immature dorsal horn circuits predominantly exhibit excitatory tone, with weaker inhibitory GABA and glycine signaling. It is uncertain whether or not this lack of inhibitory processing increases the neonate's perception of pain. Flexion reflexes may be elicited with either tactile or nociceptive touch; conversely, neonates with no behavioral reaction to heel lance showed a strongly activated cortex on EEG in one study, demonstrating the inadequacy of behavioral indicators to reliably detect pain [60].

Distinguishing between pain and agitation is also difficult as there are overlapping behavioral and physiologic manifestations [61]. Facial expression (total facial activity with specific features including brow lowering, eye squeeze, nasolabial furrow, and open mouth) is considered the most sensitive behavioral indicator of acute pain. Other behavior pain indicators include body posture, limb movements, cry, consolability, and sleep/wakefulness. Physiological parameters include heart rate, respiratory rate and pattern, oxygen saturation,

Diagnostic procedures	Arterial puncture, bronchoscopy, endoscopy, heel lancing, lumbar puncture, retinopathy of prematurity examination, suprapubic bladder tap, venipuncture
Therapeutic procedures	Bladder catheterization, central line insertion/removal, chest tube insertion/removal, chest physiotherapy, dressing change, gavage tube insertion, intramuscular injection, peripheral venous catheterization, tracheal tube insertion/removal, mechanical ventilation, tracheal suctioning, postural drainage, adhesive tape removal, ventricular tap
Surgical procedures	Circumcision
	Other surgical procedures

Table 8. Commonly performed painful procedures in the neonatal intensive care unit.

and blood pressure. These parameters are also important, but less specific, as alterations may be the result of the underlying disease process rather than pain. In the mechanically ventilated neonate with neuromuscular blocking therapy, pain must be evaluated based on changes in heart rate or blood pressure. Biological markers for pain such as emotional sweating (palm or sole, measured by skin conductance or galvanic skin response) or increased stress hormones (serum or saliva cortisol) are used in research but have limited clinical utility. Among the validated neonatal pain scales, premature infant pain profile (PIPP) assesses procedural pain, and neonatal pain, agitation, and sedation scale (N-PASS) assesses ongoing pain and sedation in both term and preterm neonates, providing an advantage over other available neonatal pain assessment tools (**Table 9**) [62–65].

5.2. Therapeutic approach

Neonatal pain is best managed using a tiered approach. Painful procedures should be avoided when possible through the use of noninvasive monitoring and bundling of laboratory blood draws. Non-pharmacological therapy, such as nonnutritive sucking, oral sucrose, breast or bottle feeding, and swaddling, can be used during mildly painful events (i.e., lab draws, line insertion, removal of adhesives, wound treatment, bladder catheterization). Topical anesthetics may be used prior to skin-breaking procedures, though caution must be exercised in the preterm neonate as the epidermis is structurally and functionally immature, increasing the risk of toxicity. Acetaminophen is effective for mild pain and as an adjuvant for moderate to severe pain. Ketamine is a potent analgesic and NMDA antagonist that can be utilized during moderate to severe painful procedures of short duration or as an adjuvant to prevent opioid tolerance. Systemic opioid analgesics are utilized to treat moderate to severe pain in conjunction with the above therapies (**Table 10**) [66, 67]. Analgesic medications are most reliable when given intravenously, as oral absorption is unpredictable in the neonate [64, 68].

Pain scale	Variables included	Type of pain assessed
Premature infant pain profile (PIPP)	Heart rate, oxygen saturation, facial actions	Procedural, postoperative
Neonatal infant pain score (NIPS)	Facial expression, crying, breathing patterns, arm/leg movement, arousal	Procedural
Neonatal facial coding system (NFCS)	Facial actions	Procedural
Neonatal pain, agitation, and sedation scale (N-PASS)	Crying, irritability, facial expression, extremity tone, vital signs	Procedural, postoperative, mechanically ventilated patients
Cry, requires oxygen, increased vital signs, expression, sleeplessness (CRIES)	Crying, facial expression, sleeplessness, requires oxygen to stay at >95% saturation, increased vital signs	Postoperative
COMFORT scale	Movement, calmness, facial tension, alertness, respiration rate, muscle tome, heart rate, blood pressure	Postoperative, critical care
Douleur Aigue du Nouveau-ne (DAN)	Facial expression, limb movements, vocal expression	Procedural

Table 9. Summary of validated neonatal pain scales.

http://dx.doi.org/10.5772/66932

Medication	Intermittent dose	Infusion dose	Adverse effects
Acetaminophen	10 mg/kg IV/PO	N/A	None reported*
NSAIDS	Not recommended	N/A	Unwanted ductal closure, gastropathy, nephropathy, NEC, IVH, surgical bleeding
Morphine	0.05–0.1 mg/kg IV	0.005–0.03 mg per hour	Respiratory depression, decreased gastrointestinal motility, hypotension, urinary retention
Fentanyl	1 mcg/kg IV	0.5–2 mcg/kg per hour	Respiratory depression, hypotension, muscle rigidity, hypothermia
Ketamine	0.5–2 mg/kg IV	0.5–1 mg/kg per hour	Respiratory depression, increased secretions

NSAIDS, nonsteroidal anti-inflammatory drugs; NEC: necrotizing enterocolitis; IVH: intraventricular hemorrhage
*No reported adverse effects at therapeutic doses. Known hepatotoxicity with overdosing.

Table 10. Recommended analgesic dosing for neonates.

Postsurgical pain should be anticipated and preemptively treated to mitigate the pain and stress response. In conjunction with analgesic medications, local anesthetics may be administered as a field block, as a targeted nerve block, or as an epidural block (**Table 11**) to effectively treat procedural and surgical pain. Care must be taken during the placement of

Block	Indications
Caudal epidural block	Lower abdominal surgery, inguinal herniorrhaphy, circumcision, orchidopexy, lower limb and pelvic orthopedic surgery
Caudal epidural catheter *	*Lumbar level*: lower abdominal, pelvic, and lower limb surgery *Thoracic level*: upper abdominal, renal, or thoracic surgery
Paravertebral block (via catheter)	Unilateral thoracic or renal surgery
Intercostal nerve blocks	Thoracic surgery, multiple levels typically required
Brachial plexus block (axillary or infraclavicular)	PICC line placement, ischemic limb salvage (arterial vasodilation)
Rectus sheath block	Umbilical/paraumbilical hernia, laparoscopic surgery, pyloromyotomy
Transversus abdominis plane (TAP) block	Lower abdominal surgery
Penile block	Circumcision
Femoral nerve block	PICC line placement lower limbs, muscle biopsy, skin graft, clubfoot repair

*Non-tunneled caudal epidural catheters should be removed after 72 hours or sooner when visible signs of soiling are present to minimize infectious risks.

Table 11. Neuraxial and peripheral nerve block indications.

local anesthetics, as unintended intravascular delivery can lead to systemic toxicity manifesting as altered consciousness, seizures, hemodynamic instability, and ultimately cardiovascular collapse. Safe practice includes aspiration prior to injection, slow incremental dosing, adherence to maximum dosing guidelines, and appropriate dose reductions for the neonate (**Table 12**) [69]. Local anesthetic toxicity must be promptly recognized and treated (**Table 13**) [70].

Local anesthetic	**Standard maximum dose ***	**Recommended neonatal dose**	**Comments**
Bupivacaine	2.5 mg/kg	1 mg/kg	Commonly used for field blocks and wound infiltration
Ropivacaine	3 mg/kg	1.5 mg/kg	Decreased motor block and cardiotoxicity compared with bupivacaine Vasoconstrictor effects (avoid using for digital and penile blocks)
Lidocaine	5 mg/kg	2.5 mg/kg	
Prilocaine	Not recommended	Not recommended	Concern for methemoglobinemia
Chloroprocaine	14 mg/kg	7 mg/kg	No plasma accumulation due to short half life
Topical anesthetic	**Maximum dose**		**Comments**
Eutectic mixture of local anesthetics (EMLA)	1 g/5 kg	1 g	Equal parts lidocaine and prilocaine Maximum skin contact 1 hour Risk of methemoglobinemia increased in premature neonates

*Maximum doses are additive and not independent of each other; *local anesthetic dosing should be decreased by 50% in neonates.*

Table 12. Commonly used local anesthetics.

Local anesthetic toxicity (LAST) management
• Obtain help
• Managing the airway, administering 100% oxygen
• Treat seizure activity (benzodiazepines preferred)
• Alert nearest facility capable of cardiopulmonary bypass
• Support cardiovascular function (prolonged CPR, reduced epinephrine doses)
• Institute 20% lipid emulsion therapy (lipidrescue.org)

Table 13. Treatment of local anesthetic toxicity.

http://dx.doi.org/10.5772/66932

Author details

Marissa Vadi*, Chelan Nour, Patrick Leiter and Harmony Carter

*Address all correspondence to: mvadi@llu.edu

Loma Linda University School of Medicine, Loma Linda, CA, USA

References

[1] Abman SH, Chatfield BA, Hall SL, McMurty IF. Role of endothelium derived relaxing factor during transition of pulmonary circulation at birth. Am J Physiol. 1990;**259**:H1921–H1927.

[2] Hagen PT, Scholz DG, Edwards WD. Incidence and size of patent foramen ovale during the first 10 decades of life: An autopsy of 965 normal hearts. Mayo Clin Proc. 1984;**59**:17–20.

[3] Robertson NRC. Perinatal physiology. In: Godfrey S, Baum JD, editors. Clinical Paediatric Physiology. London: Blackwell Scientific Publications; 1979. pp. 134–192.

[4] Rudolph AM, Heymann MA. Fetal and neonatal circulation and respiration. Annu Rev Physiol. 1974;**36**:187–207.

[5] Muller N, Volgyesi G, Bryan ME, Bryan AC. The consequences of diaphragmatic muscle fatigue in the newborn infant. J Pediatr. 1979;**95**:793–797.

[6] Keens TG, Bryan AC, Levison H, Ianuzzo CD. Developmental pattern of muscle fiber types in human ventilatory muscles. J Appl Physiol Respir Environ Exerc Physiol. 1978;**44**:909–913.

[7] Cochrane WH. Anatomy and physiology of the newborn related to anesthesia. Can Anaesth Soc J. 1961;**8**:169–176.

[8] Katz-Salamon M, Lagercrantz H. Hypoxic ventilatory defence in very preterm infants: Attenuation in long-term oxygen treatment. Arch Dis Child Fetal Neonatal Ed. 1994;**70**:F90–F95.

[9] Drukkar A, Guignard JP. Renal aspects of the term and preterm infant: A selective update. Curr Opin Pediatr. 2002;**14**:175–182.

[10] Yon JH, Daniel-Johnson J, Carter LB, Jevtovic-Todorovic V. Anesthesia induces neuronal cell death in the developing rat brain via the intrinsic and extrinsic apoptotic pathways. Neuroscience. 2005;**135**:815–827. DOI: 10.1016/j.neuroscience.2005.03.064

[11] SmartTots. Consensus Statement on the use of Anesthetic and Sedative Drugs in Infants and Toddlers [Internet]. 2015. Available from: http://smarttots.org/about/consensus-statement/ [Accessed 2016-10-17].

[12] American Society of Anesthesiologists. ASA Physical Status Classification System [Internet]. 2014. Available from: https://www.asahq.org/resources/clinical-information/asa-physical-status-classification-system [Accessed 2016-10-30].

[13] Cote CJ, Goudsouzian NG, Liu LM, Dedrick DF, Szyfelbein SK. Assessment of risk factors related to the acid aspiration syndrome in pediatric patients – gastric ph and residual volume. Anesthesiology. 1982;**56**:70–72.

[14] Apfelbaum JL, Caplan RA, Connis RT, Epstein BS, Nickinovich DG, Warner MA. Practice guidelines for preoperative fasting and the use of pharmacologic agents to reduce the risk of pulmonary aspiration: Application to healthy patients undergoing elective procedures: An updated report by the American Society of Anesthesiologists Committee on Standards and Practice Parameters. Anesthesiology. 2011;**114**:494–511. DOI: 10.1097/ALN.0b013e3181fcbfd9

[15] Warner MA, Warner ME, Warner DO, Warner LO, Warner EJ. Perioperative pulmonary aspiration in infants and children. Anesthesiology. 1999;**90**:66–71.

[16] Olsson GL, Hallen B, Hambraeus-Jonzon K. Aspiration during anaesthesia: A computer-aided study of 185,358 anaesthetics. Acta Anaesthesiol Scand. 1986;**30**:84–92.

[17] Walker RW. Pulmonary aspiration in pediatric anesthetic practice in the UK: A prospective survey of specialist pediatric centers over a one-year period. Paediatr Anaesth. 2013;**23**:702–711.

[18] Borland LM, Sereika SM, Woelfel SK, Saitz EW, Carrillo PA, Lupin JL, Motoyama EK. Pulmonary aspiration in pediatric patients during general anesthesia: Incidence and outcome. J Clin Anesth. 1998;**10**:95–102.

[19] Krane EJ, Haberkern CM, Jacobson LE. Postoperative apnea, bradycardia, and oxygen desaturation in formerly premature infants: Prospective comparison of spinal and general anesthesia. Anesth Analg. 1995;**80**:7–13.

[20] Sale SM, Read JA, Stoddart PA, Wolf AR. Prospective comparison of sevoflurane and desflurane in formerly premature infants undergoing inguinal herniotomy. Br J Anaesth. 2006;**96**:774–778. DOI: 10.1093/bja/ael100

[21] Davidson AJ, Morton NS Arnup SJ, de Graaff JC, Disma N, Withington DE, Frawley G, Hunt RW, Hardy P, Khotcholava M, von Ungern Sternberg BS, Wilton N, Tuo P, Salvo I, Ormond G, Stargatt R, Locatelli BG, McCann ME. Apnea after awake regional and general anesthesia in infants: The general anesthesia compared to spinal anesthesia study–comparing apnea and neurodevelopmental outcomes, a randomized controlled trial. Anesthesiology. 2015;**123**:38–54. DOI: 10.1097/ALN.0000000000000709

[22] Cote CJ, Zaslavsky A, Downes JJ, Kurth CD, Welborn LG, Warner LO, Malviya SV. Postoperative apnea in former preterm infants after inguinal herniorrhaphy. A combined analysis. Anesthesiology. 1995;**82**:809–822.

[23] Kelly DH, Shannon DC. Treatment of apnea and excessive periodic breathing in the full-term infant. Pediatrics. 1981;**68**:183–186.

[24] American Society of Anesthesiologists. Standards for Basic Anesthetic Monitoring [Internet]. 2015. Available from: http://www.asahq.org/~/media/sites/asahq/files/public/resources/standards-guidelines/standards-for-basic-anesthetic-monitoring.pdf [Accessed 2016-08-01].

[25] Taneja B, Srivastava V, Saxena KN. Physiological and anaesthetic considerations for the preterm neonate undergoing surgery. J Neonatal Surg. 2012;**1**:14.

[26] Hillier SC, Krishna G, Brasoveanu E. Neonatal anesthesia. Semin Pediatr Surg. 2004;**13**:142–151. DOI: 10.1053/j.sempedsurg.2004.04.002

[27] Pani N, Panda CK. Anaesthetic consideration for neonatal surgical emergencies. Indian J Anaesth. 2012;**56**:463–469. DOI: 10.4103/0019-5049.103962

[28] Schindler E, Kowald B, Suess H, Niehaus-Borquez B, Tausch B, Brecher A. Catheterization of the radial or brachial artery in neonates and infants. Paediatr Anaesth. 2005;**15**:677–682. DOI: 10.1111/j.1460-9592.2004.01522.x

[29] Freeman JJ, Gadepalli SK, Siddiqui SM, Jarboe MD, Hirschi RB. Improving central line infection rates in the neonatal intensive care unit: Effect of hospital location, site of insertion, and implementation of catheter-associated bloodstream infection protocols. J Pediatr Surg. 2015;**50**:860–863. DOI: 10.1016/j.jpedsurg.2015.02.001

[30] Lerman J, Sikich N, Kleinman S, Yentis S. The pharmacology of sevoflurane in infants and children. Anesthesiology. 1994;**80**:814–824.

[31] Taylor RH, Lerman J. Minimum alveolar concentration of desflurane and hemodynamic responses in neonates, infants, and children. Anesthesiology. 1991;**75**:975–979.

[32] Cameron CB, Robinson S, Gregory GA. The minimum anesthetic concentration of isoflurane in children. Anesth Analg. 1984;**63**:418–420.

[33] Cote CJ, Lerman J, Anderson BJ, editors. A Practice of Anesthesia for Infants and Children. 5th ed. Philadephia: Elsevier Saunders; 2013. 111 p. DOI: 10.1213/ane.0b013e3182a00428

[34] Pittaway A. Principles of anaesthesia for term neonates: An updated practical guide. Anaesth Intensive Care. 2011;**12**:95–98. DOI: 10.1016/j.mpaic.2010.11.002

[35] Davis PJ, Cladis FP, Motoyama EK, editors. Smith's Anesthesia for Infants and Children. 8th ed. Philadelphia: Elsevier Mosby; 2011. pp. 192–195. DOI: 10.1016/c2009-0-49104-9

[36] Brandom BW, Fine GF. Neuromuscular blocking drugs in pediatric anesthesia. Anesthesiol Clin North America. 2002;**20**:45–58. DOI: 10.1016/S0889-8537(03)00054-3

[37] Micromedex. Succinylcholine Chloride [Internet]. 2016. Available from: http://www.micromedexsolutions.com/micromedex2/librarian/CS/A5B83B/ND_PR/evidencexpert/ND_P/evidencexpert/DUPLICATIONSHIELDSYNC/392347/ND_PG/evidencexpert/ND_B/evidencexpert/ND_AppProduct/evidencexpert/ND_T/evidencexpert/PFActionId/evidencexpert.DoIntegratedSearch?SearchTerm=succinylcholine# [Accessed 2016-09-01].

[38] Engelhardt T. Rapid sequence induction has no use in pediatric anesthesia. Paediatr Anaesth. 2015;**25**:5–8. DOI: 10.1111/pan.12544

[39] Won YJ, Lim BG, Lee DK, Kim H, Kong MH, Lee IO. Sugammadex for reversal of rocuronium-induced neuromuscular blockade in pediatric patients: A systematic review and meta-analysis. Medicine (Baltimore). 2016;**95**:e4678. DOI: 10.1097/MD.0000000000004678

[40] Bailey AG, McNaull PP, Jooste E, Tuchman JB. Perioperative crystalloid and colloid fluid management in children: Where are we and how did we get here? Anesth Analg. 2010;**110**:375–390. DOI: 10.1213/ANE.0b013e3181b6b3b5

[41] Arya VK. Basics of fluid and blood transfusion therapy in paediatric surgical patients. Indian J Anaesth. 2012;**56**:454–462. DOI: 10.4103/0019-5049.103960

[42] Boldt J. Use of albumin: An update. Br J Anaesth. 2010;**104**:276–284. DOI: 10.1093/bja/aep393

[43] Uhing MR. The albumin controversy. Clin Perinatol. 2004;**31**:475–488.

[44] Gray R. Which colloid to choose for neonates, infants and children. South Afr J Anaesth Analg. 2015;**21**:56–58.

[45] Cote CJ, Lerman J, Anderson BJ, editors. A Practice of Anesthesia for Infants and Children. 5th ed. Philadephia: Elsevier Saunders; 2013. 198 p. DOI: 10.1213/ane.0b013e3182a00428

[46] Davies P, Robertson S, Hegde S, Greenwood R, Massey E, Davis P. Calculating the required transfusion volume in children. Transfusion. 2007;**47**:212–216.

[47] Keir AK, Stanworth SJ. Neonatal plasma transfusion: An evidence-based review. Transfus Med Rev. 2016;**30**:174–182. DOI: 10.1016/j.tmrv.2016.07.001

[48] Sloan SR, Parker RI. Current status of platelet transfusion in pediatric patients. Transfus Med Rev. 2016;**30**:230–234. DOI: 10.1016/j.tmrv.2016.07.006

[49] Goel R, Cushing MM, Tobian AA. Pediatric patient blood management programs: Not just transfusing little adults. Transfus Med Rev. 2016;**30**:235–241. DOI: 10.1016/j.tmrv.2016.07.004

[50] International Association for the Study of Pain. IASP Taxonomy [Internet]. 2012. Available from: http://www.iasp-pain.org/Taxonomy#Pain [Accessed: 2016-09-07].

[51] Anand KJ, Sippell WG, Aynsley-Green A. Randomised trial of fentanyl anaesthesia in preterm babies undergoing surgery: Effects on the stress response. Lancet. 1987;**1**:62–66. DOI: 10.1016/S0140-6736(87)90065-1

[52] Anand KJ, Hickey PR. Pain and its effects in the human neonate and fetus. N Engl J Med. 1987;**317**:1321–1329. DOI: 10.1056/NEJM198711193172105

[53] Rutter N, Doyal D. Neonatal care and management of pain: Historical and ethical issues. Semin Neonatol. 1998;**3**:297–302. DOI: 10.1016/S1084-2756(98)80084-5

[54] Anand KJ, International Evidence-Based Group for Neonatal Pain. Consensus statement for the prevention and management of pain in the newborn. Arch Pediatr Adolesc Med. 2001;**155**:173–180. DOI: 10.1001/archpedi.155.2.173

[55] Anand KJ, Scalzo FM. Can adverse neonatal experiences alter brain development and subsequent behavior? Biol Neonate. 2000; **77**:69–82. DOI: 10.1159/000014197

[56] Montirosso R, Casini E, Del Prete A, Zanini R, Bellu R, Borgatti R, NEO-ACQUA Study Group. Neonatal developmental care in infant pain management and internalizing behaviours at 18 months in prematurely born children. Eur J Pain. 2016;**20**:1010–1021. DOI: 10.1002/ejp.826

[57] Grunau RE, Holsti L, Haley DW, Oberlander T, Weinberg J, Solimano A, Whitfield MF, Fitzgerald C, Yu W. Neonatal procedural pain exposure predicts lower cortisol and behavioral reactivity in preterm infants in the NICU. Pain. 2005;**113**:293–300. DOI: 10.1016/j.pain.2004.10.020

[58] Victoria NC, Murphy AZ. Exposure to early life pain: Long term consequences and contributing mechanisms. Curr Opin Behav Sci. 2016;**7**:61–68. DOI: 10.1016/j.cobeha.2015.11.015

[59] Victoria NC, Murphy AZ. The long-term impact of early life pain on adult responses to anxiety and stress: Historical perspectives and empirical evidence. Exp Neurol. 2016;**275**:261–273. DOI: 10.1016/j.expneurol.2015.07.017

[60] Fitzgerald M. What do we really know about newborn infant pain? Exp Physiol. 2015;**100**:1451–1457. DOI: 10.1113/EP085134

[61] Maxwell LG, Malavolta CP, Fraga MV. Assessment of pain in the neonate. Clin Perinatol. 2013;**40**:457–469. DOI: 10.1016/j.clp.2013.05.001

[62] Hummel P, van Dijk M. Pain assessment: Current status and challenges. Semin Fetal Neonatal Med. 2006;**11**:237–245. DOI: 10.1016/j.siny.2006.02.004

[63] Ballantyne M, Stevens B, McAllister M, Dionne K, Jack A. Validation of the premature infant pain profile in the clinical setting. Clin J Pain. 1999;**15**:297–303.

[64] Witt N, Coynor S, Edwards C, Bradshaw H. A guide to pain assessment and management in the neonate. Curr Emerg Hosp Med Rep. 2016;**4**:1–10. DOI: 10.1007/s40138-016-0089-y

[65] Hillman BA, Tabrizi MN, Gauda EB, Carson KA, Aucott SW. The neonatal pain, agitation and sedation scale and the bedside nurse's assessment of neonates. J Perinatol. 2015;**35**:128–131. DOI: 10.1038/jp.2014.154

[66] Morton NS. Local and regional anaesthesia in infants. Contin Educ Anaesth Crit Care Pain. 2004;**4**:148–151. DOI: 10.1093/bjaceaccp/mkh041

[67] Bosenberg A, Flick RP. Regional anesthesia in neonates and infants. Clin Perinatol. 2013; **40**:525–538. DOI: 10.1016/j.clp.2013.05.011

[68] Anand KJ, Aranda JV, Berde CB, Buckman S, Capparelli EV, Carlo WA, Hummel P, Lantos J, Johnston CC, Lehr VT, Lynn AM, Maxwell LG, Oberlander TF, Raju TN, Soriano SG, Walco GA. Analgesia and anesthesia for neonates: Study design and ethical issues. Clin Ther. 2005;**27**:814–843. DOI: 10.1016/j.clinthera.2005.06.021

[69] Gunter JB. Benefit and risks of local anesthetics in infants and children. Paediatr Drugs. 2002;**4**:649–672.

[70] American Society of Regional Anesthesia and Pain Medicine. Checklist for Treatment of Local Anesthetic Systemic Toxicity [Internet]. 2016. Available from: https://www.asra.com/advisory-guidelines/article/3/checklist-for-treatment-of-local-anesthetic-systemic-toxicity [Accessed: 2016-10-30].

Chapter 3

Spinal Anaesthetic Management in Paediatric Surgery

Esra Caliskan

Additional information is available at the end of the chapter

http://dx.doi.org/10.5772/67409

Abstract

The first paediatric cases involving the use of spinal anaesthesia were published at the end of the nineteenth century. However, the technique did not receive much interest in paediatric anaesthesia until the 1980s. In the last three decades, paediatric spinal anaesthesia has received widespread approval as an alternative technique to general anaesthesia in school-/preschool-aged children, particularly in term and preterm neonates with high risk associated with general anaesthesia. The development of new and safer local anaesthetics mainly through better understanding of the pharmacokinetics and dynamics and dedicated paediatric tools are the keys to this success. Paediatric spinal anaesthesia is an easy and effective technique, and its high efficiency and safety are supported by the presence of numerous publications from the medical literature. However, it remains limited to situations in which general anaesthesia poses a major risk. Despite these advances, it is important to understand the correct technique and the anatomy of children at different ages. Also, the appropriate equipment, the pharmacokinetics and toxicities of local anaesthetics and the indications and complications of paediatric regional blocks should be well known. The goal of this chapter is to review and discuss some of these topics of paediatric spinal anaesthesia for paediatric surgery.

Keywords: paediatrics, anaesthetic techniques, regional anaesthesia, paediatric spinal anaesthesia, complications, anaesthetic management

1. Introduction

1.1. History of paediatric spinal anaesthesia

The use of paediatric regional anaesthesia began in the first half of the 1900s. In 1898, Bier [1] performed the first spinal anaesthetic, and two of his patients were children. Bier's publications were followed by reports by Donitz in Europe [2]. In addition, in 1909–1910, two detailed articles about more than 100 children with spinal anaesthesia were published by Gray [3, 4] in the Lancet.

With the development of general anaesthesia, there was little interest in paediatric spinal anaesthesia until the 1950s. Since then, paediatric spinal anaesthesia has become a more popular technique for the anaesthesiologist, and during the last three decades, the spinal anaesthetic approach has increased dramatically in children. This technique has been used safely in premature and ex-premature infants with a high risk of apnoea associated with general anaesthesia [5–8]. Also, spinal anaesthesia is an uncomplicated and effective technique that provides a rapid onset and exceedingly effective analgesia, sympathetic and motor block in the lower part of the body [9].

Despite the increased prevalence of spinal anaesthesia in children, it is still not practised everywhere owing to the use of conventional general anaesthesia.

2. Spinal anaesthetic approach: anatomical and physiological differences in paediatric patients

2.1. Anatomical structure of and differences in vertebral column

The anatomical structure of the spinal column in children differs from that of adults. In premature infants (approximately 90%), the spinal cord terminates between the L2–L3 vertebra [10]. In newborns, the spinal cord extends down to the level of the L3 lumbar vertebra, compared with the L1 lumbar vertebra in adults (**Figure 1**) [11–13].

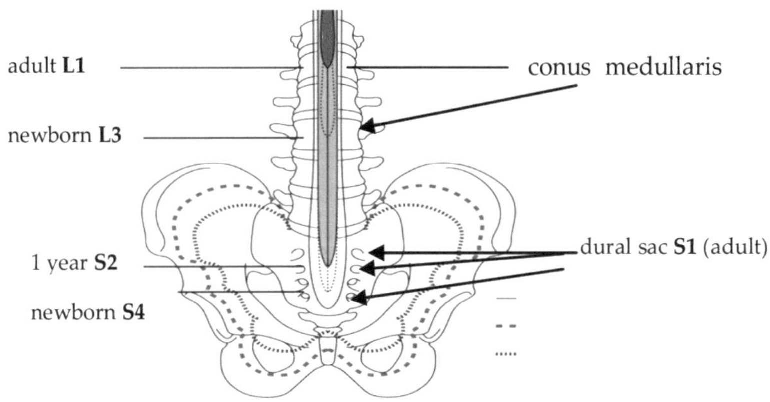

Figure 1. Anatomical structure and differences between paediatric and adult invertebral column (Remodified from Frawley and Ingelmo [13]).

The dural sac ends at the L4 vertebra at birth but reaches S2 by the end of the first year of life (**Figure 1**) [13]. Shin et al. confirmed that the end of the dural sac was at a median level of the upper S2 in children aged less than 36 months of age [14].

The iliac crest (intercristal line—Tuffier's line) can be used to determine safe puncture levels for children in the same way as in adults. In infants, the intercristal line passes through the vertebral column at the L4–5 or L5–S1 interspace, well below the termination of the spinal cord [13]. Therefore, the L4–5 or L5–S1 intervertebral space should be used for needle placement in children.

Studies related to vertebral anatomy in children demonstrated that the distance between the skin and the subarachnoid space at the level of the L4–5 interspace is 6 mm at birth and 10–12 mm at 1 year of age [15]. Ecoffey et al. [16] reported that the distance between the skin and the subarachnoid space was 10–18 mm in the lumbar region and 7–14 mm in the thoracic region in children less than 3 years of age.

The pelvis has a more rounded structure in infants, and the iliac crest is lower than in adults. Another anatomical difference in paediatric patients is the flexibility of a child's spine and intervertebral spaces, which are easily palpated [13]. In addition to these characteristics, ossification of the vertebral lamina is incomplete, and the spinal needle can readily enter the bone. The lumbar spinal canal differs in the paediatric age group too; the interpedicular diameter of the spinal canal at the lumbar level is quite wide and is 70% of the adult size at birth [9, 17].

All these anatomical differences between children and adult scan facilitate dural puncture in children, but paediatric spinal anaesthesia is a specialised technique, and these anatomical characteristics must be taken into consideration in order not to cause complications when performing the spinal technique.

2.2. Physiological differences between adult and paediatric patients

In neonates, insufficient myelinisation and a weak endoneurium provide an ineffective barrier to drug diffusion. These anatomical and physiological characteristics mean the rapid onset and offset of block [12, 18].

Vascularisation of the pia mater is relatively high in neonates. Cardiac output is also higher in children than in adults. Because of these two factors, local anaesthetic reabsorption is rapid, and the duration of block is shorter. Compared to adults, the total cerebrospinal fluid (CSF) volume is higher in children (neonates, 10 ml kg^{-1}; infants and toddlers, 4 ml kg^{-1}), and because the ligament density is low, the feeling of loss of resistance is less marked than in adults.

In infants, the lack of lumbar lordosis and increased limits of spinal flexibility can predispose to high spinal blockade with differences in positioning compared with older children [12, 13].

3. Benefits of spinal anaesthesia in children

3.1. Effective pain control

Spinal anaesthesia provides effective analgesia with minimal physiological changes or adverse effects and is an alternative to systemic analgesics (such as opioid and non-opioid analgesics) [19]. This feature provides a significant advantage in cases where systemic opioid use is contraindicated, especially in children at risk of opioid-induced adverse effects.

Effective analgesia also creates ideal physiological conditions for the recovery period for children and their families. An awake, cooperative and painless child adjusts more easily to the postoperative period. Additionally, efficient pain control reduces adverse effects due to the neuroendocrine stress response.

3.2. The effects of anaesthetics on neuronal development

In recent years, many important studies and preclinical data have been reported that describe how general anaesthesia affects neurodevelopmental outcome in young animals [20]. Changes in brain development include dose-dependent neuronal apoptosis, impairment of neuronal differentiation, synaptogenesis and changes to dendritic morphology [21].

The neurodegenerative effect seems to be both time and dose dependent. In animal studies, anaesthetic drugs (these act through the NMDA and GABA receptors) played a role in neurodegeneration.

In young animals, long-term cognitive and behavioural changes associated with general anaesthetics have been shown in several studies, but these findings must be supported by human studies and clinical data.

In recent years, various reviews, cohort studies and two meta-analyses have established that there is an association between anaesthesia in childhood and neurodevelopmental outcome [22].

In a randomised clinical trial, Davidson et al. compared the neurodevelopmental outcome in children who received either awake regional anaesthesia or sevorane-based general anaesthesia for inguinal herniorrhaphy in early infancy (the general anaesthesia compared to spinal anaesthesia (GAS) trial) [23]. The authors found that exposure to just less than 1 h sevoflurane general anaesthesia in infancy did not increase the risk of adverse neurodevelopmental outcome at 2 years of age. Nonetheless, reducing exposure to general anaesthesia especially in premature infants is important so as to reduce the deleterious effects of inhalational anaesthesia.

4. Physiological effects and advantages of spinal anaesthesia

4.1. Respiratory effects

Spinal anaesthesia has been correlated with minimal respiratory changes and ensures continuity of spontaneous breathing during surgery. This advantage is important in high-risk children in whom the anaesthetist wishes to avoid tracheal intubation and mechanical ventilation.

In summary, the respiratory benefits of spinal anaesthesia are as follows: effective analgesia without respiratory depression, improved respiratory performance and enhanced ventilatory response to hypercapnia with bupivacaine (possible mechanism is a direct stimulating effect of bupivacaine on the respiratory centre) [24].

In the neonatal period, the risk of opioid-related respiratory depression and sensitivity to muscle relaxant is more pronounced. However, spinal anaesthesia decreases the requirement for anaesthetic agents, muscle relaxants and opioids during surgery. These effects are especially important for reducing the risk of postoperative apnoea in high-risk infants that require surgery in this period [25].

4.2. Haemodynamic properties

Spinal anaesthesia in infants and young children is characterised by remarkable haemodynamic stability [15, 19, 26]. This physiological feature can be expressed clinically as the lack of significant decreases in blood pressure and the reduced need for volume preloading or vasoconstrictor use. This property is important especially in the neonatal period. The neonatal heart is immature immediately after birth and in the first month of life. Myocardial compliance and contractility are lower than in adults. This means that the ability to cope with stress with afterload is also reduced [27]. Therefore, especially in infants with congenital cardiac disease, spinal anaesthesia should be the preferred anaesthetic approach as it has minimum cardio-depressant effects.

Haemodynamic stability during spinal anaesthesia in infants can be considered as one of the advantages of spinal anaesthesia [28, 29]. Because of this feature, awake spinal anaesthesia is usually regarded as safe in high-risk infants [15].

4.3. Neuroendocrine stress response

Neuroendocrine stress responses associated with surgical trauma cause some hormonal changes in plasma. Increased levels of plasma cortisol and suppression of anabolic hormones, such as insulin, cause harmful effects during the perioperative period [30]. As a result, postoperative pain associated with surgical trauma may cause instability in haemodynamic parameters, behavioural changes and neuroendocrine stress responses [31, 32].

Regional anaesthesia can reduce the stress response associated with surgical trauma (6–10). Many studies have confirmed this [30, 33]. Wolf et al. [34] reported that, in infants undergoing major surgery, central block with epidural anaesthesia was more efficacious than high-dose opioid in suppressing cardiovascular and stress responses. The same authors also pointed out that high spinal anaesthesia is more effective than intermittently delivered epidural anaesthesia to reduce stress responses to surgery [35].

The neuroendocrine stress response is a phenomenon induced by surgical trauma. Severe stress may be pathological and may increase postoperative morbidity and mortality. Spinal anaesthesia is an effective method for attenuating the surgical stress response and may be considered an alternative to general anaesthesia especially in immunocompromised or malnourished paediatric patients [26].

4.4. Gastrointestinal function

Expected effects of opioid drugs are increased intestinal muscle tone and a slowdown in peristalsis [36]. This situation is particularly undesirable in necrotising enterocolitis and gastroschisis surgery in the neonatal period, because it may lead to anastomotic leak after surgery. However, spinal anaesthesia is associated with earlier return of gastrointestinal function. The vasodilator effect of autonomic blockade increases splanchnic perfusion and peristalsis. Early recovery of bowel movements favours early recovery of appetite, eating and discharge from hospital.

5. Indications and contraindications of spinal anaesthesia

5.1. Indications

Operations associated with the lower part of the body include abdominal (e.g. exploratory laparotomy, pyloromyotomy, omphalocele and gastroschisis and inguinal hernia repair), urological (hypospadias, orchiopexy and circumcision) and orthopaedic surgery and constitute the main indications for spinal anaesthesia (**Table 1**) [9, 37].

General surgical procedures

Abdominal pathologies

- Gastroschisis
- Omphalocele
- Exploratory laparotomy
- Colostomy
- Appendectomy
- Pyloromyotomy

Inguinal and umbilical herniorrhaphy

Lower extremity procedures and orthopaedic surgery

- Club foot repair
- Open and closed reduction of hip
- Tumour resection
- Amputation
- Muscle biopsy

Urological surgery

- Circumcision
- Orchidopexy
- Cystoscopy
- Hydrocelectomy
- Hypospadias repair
- Vesicostomy
- Urethral reconstructive surgery

http://dx.doi.org/10.5772/67409

Other procedures

- Cardiothoracic procedures: noninvasive and invasive techniques (atrial/ventricular septal defect closure, patent ductus arteriosus ligation, etc.)
- Neurosurgical procedure: meningomyelocele operation
- Outpatient procedure: radiation oncological processes

Table 1. Indications of paediatric spinal anaesthesia.

Paediatric patients, especially premature and ex-premature infants, may require surgical interventions for several reasons in early stages of their life. In the past 30–40 years, spinal anaesthesia has been introduced to the modern surgical era as an important and suitable technique for selected surgery in high-risk premature and ex-premature infants (**Figure 2**). The use of the spinal anaesthetic approach is supported by studies in high-risk infants published by Abajian et al. [38] in 1984.

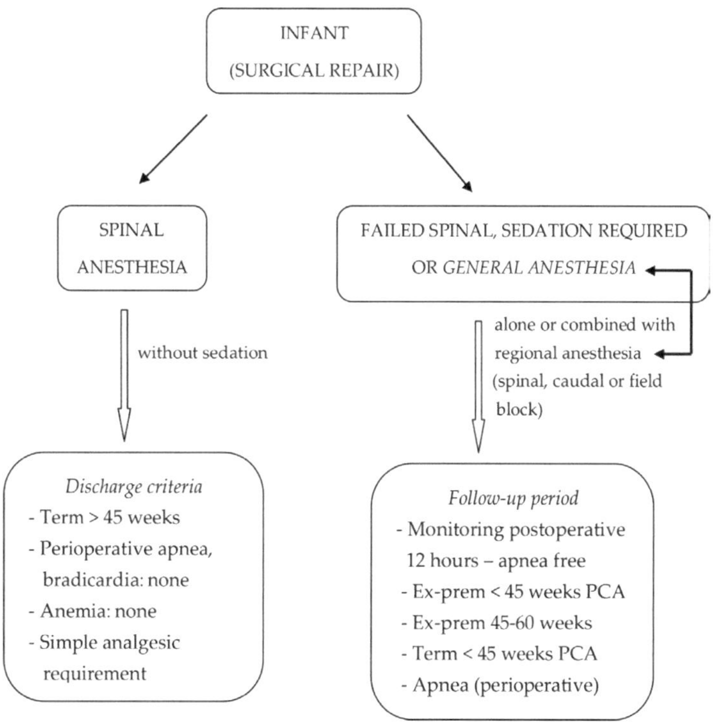

Figure 2. Chart of follow-up period after surgical intervention in infants. PCA, postconceptional age (Remodified from Frawley and Ingelmo [13] and Williams et al. [25]). Infants with pre-existing apnea and less than 45 weeks PCA are at the risk of postoperative apnea and should be kept under observation for at least postoperative 12 h.

Spinal anaesthesia is particularly important for reducing the risk of postoperative apnoea in high-risk infants and avoiding intraoperative sedation. In some specific cases, general anaesthesia may be technically difficult or associated with increased morbidity and mortality (such as in children with a known difficult airway, upper respiratory tract infection, full stomach, etc.). In such situations, spinal anaesthesia constitutes a more viable alternative for many anaesthetists.

Airway manipulation with endotracheal tube or supraglottic airway devices may not be performed in patients with a difficult airway. Likewise, in children with upper respiratory tract infection, continuous airway hyperreactivity in early stages and endotracheal intubation can cause serious respiratory complications [39]. In both cases, the spinal anaesthetic technique provides reliable airway management without endotracheal intubation and the use of a muscle relaxant. However, in such situations, if sedation is needed, special attention should be given to keeping the airway open.

Children with congenital muscular disease or respiratory muscle weakness are candidates for spinal anaesthesia. This is because general anaesthesia is thought to worsen respiratory function in the presence of muscle or pulmonary disease [11].

Spinal anaesthesia is also suitable in children with a full stomach and those who need emergency surgery, such as acute trauma patients. The risk of aspiration is less than in general anaesthesia because airway reflexes are protected during spinal anaesthesia. Nausea and vomiting are also less likely.

Paediatric patients with congenital heart disease (CHD) frequently undergo noncardiac surgical procedures for the management of both comorbidities and additional congenital anomalies [40]. Spinal anaesthesia is also used for noncardiac surgery in these paediatric patients.

Shenkman et al. and Kachko et al. [15, 41] have reported studies and experiences with spinal anaesthesia in children with congenital heart disease. Researchers consider that spinal anaesthesia is a safe and effective anaesthetic and analgesic technique in patients with CHD especially neonatal period.

In addition, studies that compared general anaesthesia with spinal anaesthesia indicated that spinal anaesthesia is associated with a significant degree of cardiorespiratory stability, a low incidence of respiratory complications and need for postoperative ventilator support and a shorter hospital stay [42].

5.1.1. Spinal anaesthesia for day-case surgery

Nowadays, another reason for preferring regional anaesthesia is its lower cost compared with general anaesthesia. Elective surgery including lower abdominal procedures can be performed as day-case surgery in paediatric patients. Spinal anaesthesia has significant advantages in outpatient surgery. These advantages include a rapid onset and recovery after surgery, the short duration of block with a single injection, easy application in experienced hands, the ability to eat sooner with a lower incidence of postoperative nausea and vomiting and early discharge from hospital.

Spinal anaesthesia is a suitable technique for the surgeries mentioned above in children from 6 months of age. Children can be discharged the same day after spinal anaesthesia depending on the discharge criteria (such as walking unassisted after spinal anaesthesia, no pain, tolerating clear fluids orally, no nausea and vomiting). However, syndromic infants and children with a history of apnoea or respiratory problems should not be discharged on the day of surgery.

5.2. Contraindications

As previously mentioned, paediatric spinal anaesthesia is a technique that is easily attempted in experienced hands. However, in addition to the indication for spinal anaesthesia, every anaesthesiologist dealing with paediatric spinal anaesthesia must have sufficient knowledge about the absolute and relative contraindications and limitations.

Absolute contraindications of spinal anaesthesia
• Infection at the puncture site
• Coagulation disorder
• Septicaemia and bacteraemia
• Axonal degenerative disease
• Severe hypovolemia
• Local anaesthetic allergy
Relative contraindications of spinal anaesthesia
• Major deformities of spinal column
• Long duration surgical procedures
• Minor abnormalities of the coagulation profile

Table 2. Absolute and relative contraindications of spinal anaesthesia.

Contraindications for spinal anaesthesia include absolute and relative contraindications [9, 43] and are listed in **Table 2**.

In addition to these contraindications, dermatological problems that prevent the sterilisation of the puncture site are also absolute contraindications [11].

Bleeding disorders and coagulopathy are comparatively rare in children, and drugs affecting coagulation function are rarely used in paediatric patients. Cases of neuroaxial haematomas have been reported after epidural anaesthesia and diagnostic lumbar puncture [44]. Therefore, the patient should be questioned about the family history for major coagulation disorders before administering spinal anaesthesia.

6. Technique

As explained in the section on anatomical structure, the anatomical configuration of the vertebra and spinal canal in paediatric patients differs from that in adults, and these differences must be taken into consideration when performing spinal anaesthesia.

Spinal anaesthesia is usually performed with the patient on their side with their back flexed and neck extended (**Figure 3**).

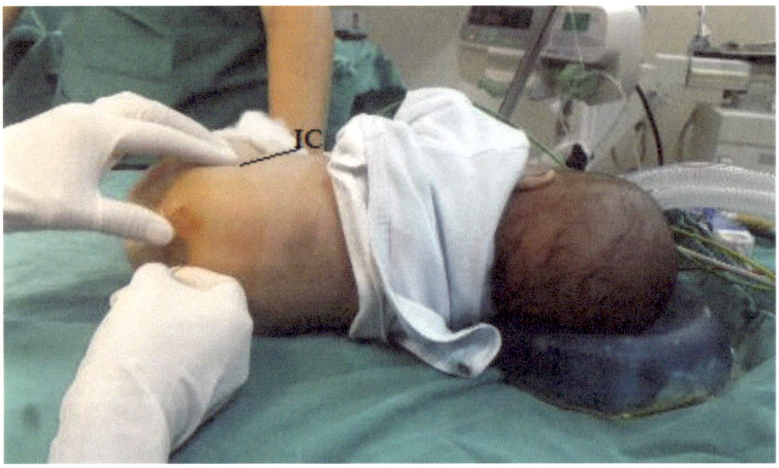

Figure 3. Lumbar puncture in the infant shown is the lateral decubitus position. In this position, puncture performed with the patient on their side with their back flexed and the neck extended for airway patency. IC, iliac crest.

The sitting position is also used in newborns and infants, but excessive flexion of the neck should be avoided [9, 45].

In children, the skin-spinal space distance is short [11]. Gupta and Saha emphasised that the depth of insertion at L4–5 level varies with age (in newborns, 10–15 mm; up to 5 years, 15–25 mm; 5–8 years, 30–40 mm) [12]. Due to the anatomical configuration of the dural sac and spinal cord in children, it is sensible to be cautious and use a low approach (L4–5 or L4–S1) (below the intercristal line) to avoid damage to the spinal cord.

To increase the success rate of the block and decrease post-puncture complications, during the puncture the spinal needle must be parallel to the dural fibre. Incorrect needle position can cause injection of local anaesthetic drug into the subdural space. This situation may give rise to an incomplete block. Before injecting local anaesthetic drug, free flow and aspiration of CSF should always be confirmed [11, 41].

After free CSF flow is observed, the needle should be forwarded by no more than 1 mm (to avoid subdural injection). Previous studies proposed that the needle be left in position for a few seconds after local anaesthetic injection. Kokki suggested that this approach would prevent the drug from tracing back into the tissues and skin puncture [38, 43]. Injection should be performed slowly over at least 20 sec.

After injecting the local anaesthetic, it is recommended that the needle should be withdrawn by reinserting a stylet. This manoeuvre reduces the formation of large hole in the dura mater. Thereby, local anaesthetic leakage is prevented at the puncture site, which is especially important in young children. Following an intrathecal injection, the lower extremity should not be moved. and the Trendelenburg position should be avoided.

Different types and lengths of spinal needle have been described for use in paediatric patients (gauge; tip design, cutting/pencil point; length, long/short). Various lengths of spinal needle are available for infants and small children, ranging from 25–50 mm [12]. A short needle allows comfortable movement and provides a minimal dead space; in infants, 25–38 mm needles are sufficiently long, and 50 mm needles are suitable in small children. In school-aged children, a standard length adult spinal needle can be used with a high success rate. In recent years, new atraumatic paediatric spinal needles have been manufactured (e.g. 26 G atraumatic needle and 27 G pencil-point needle).

The anatomical configuration of the spinal column is flatter in young children than in adults. Because of this, local anaesthetic injected into the subarachnoid space rapidly reaches the mid-thoracic level. In small children, care needs to be taken over the use of the introducer needle, because there is a short skin-spinal distance [46].

Needle type and the incidence of complications will be discussed in detail in the section on post-puncture complications. It is considered that short and thin spinal needles (e.g. 26 gauge atraumatic needle and 27 gauge pencil-point needle) significantly reduce postdural puncture complications in comparison with 22 gauge needle [11].

Kokki et al. showed that spinal puncture was successful when using cutting and pencil-point needles, with no differences between these needles in terms of post-puncture complications. Apiliogullari et al. reported that when compared with a 26 G cutting-point needle, the 27 G pencil-point needle leads to a significantly lower incidence of PDPH in children [47].

Almost half of the total CSF volume is in the spinal subarachnoid space in children. This factor plays an important role in calculating the dose of spinal blocks, with infants requiring higher volumes based on weight. The CSF in a neonate quickly dilutes the local anaesthetic after injection. This feature is one of the reasons for the use of high doses of local anaesthetic and the shorter duration of action of spinal blocks than in adults [48].

6.1. Sedation

Procedural sedation is often used in children before performing spinal anaesthesia. The aim of the sedation is to provide anxiolysis and ensure that the child remains motionless during lumbar puncture. Movement during puncture may cause injuries in neurovascular structures. Sedative drugs (such as midazolam, propofol or ketamine) may be used in small incremental doses in children. Nevertheless, Sale reported that these sedative agents and the older inhalational anaesthetics used with spinal anaesthesia seem to be associated with apnoeic episodes in neonates [49]. Newer and short-acting inhalational agents (such as sevoflurane and desflurane) seem to be safer than older ones [11, 12].

Sedative agents should be avoided as much as possible in high-risk neonates. Abajian et al. [38] described an unsupplemented spinal anaesthesia technique in ex-premature infants undergoing herniotomy in 1984. In any case, spinal anaesthesia may be used without simultaneous sedation in this high-risk group. Further studies showed that awake spinal anaesthesia reduces the risk of apnoea in newborns [7, 25].

However, except in high-risk neonates, in many children spinal anaesthesia is performed under premedication or light sedation. In addition to the previously mentioned agents, dexmedetomidine (a potent, selective alpha-2 adrenoceptor agonist) may also be used. Dexmedetomidine provides natural sleep, anxiolysis and analgesia [50].

Transdermal local anaesthetic (such as EMLA cream) can be used on the puncture area 45–60 min before lumbar puncture.

When under sedation, close monitoring should be performed for patient's safety. Standard parameters should be monitored (especially oxygenation with pulse oximetry, end-tidal carbon dioxide monitoring of respiratory function and electrocardiogram).

6.2. Local anaesthetic agents

The pharmacokinetics and pharmacodynamic characteristics of local anaesthetics (LA) alter with age. Local anaesthetics that primarily bind to plasma protein (such as bupivacaine and levobupivacaine) undergo enzymatic degradation in the liver [51, 52]. Local anaesthetics should be used carefully, particularly in infants less than 6 months of age, because they lack the ability to distribute the drug and have limited metabolism [51].

Ester-type local anaesthetics such as tetracaine and chloroprocaine are metabolised by plasma cholinesterase [9]. Aminobenzoic acid which metabolises to ester-type local anaesthetic is responsible for allergic reactions. However, allergic reactions are rare in amino-amide group local anaesthetics [9].

As well as the onset time and duration of action of regional block, the safety profile of an agent is among the factors that play a role in the choice of local anaesthetic. Tetracaine, bupivacaine, ropivacaine and levobupivacaine are still the most commonly used local anaesthetics in children [9, 47, 53–55].

Age and body weight form the basis for local anaesthetic dose calculation. Nowadays, obesity is a common problem in children. In clinical practice, the dose of local anaesthetics should be calculated according to the ideal body weight of the child [9]. Local anaesthetics can be used in different concentrations in paediatric patients.

Kokki et al. investigated the effects of local anaesthetic baricity on the block characteristics, comparing isobaric and hyperbaric bupivacaine in children. They found that the block characteristics were similar for both drugs.

In recent years, various studies on higher local anaesthetic doses for neonates (e.g. ropivacaine and levobupivacaine at a dose of 1.2 mg kg^{-1}) have been reported, but there are few data regarding the safety of this dose profile [53]. Recommended dosages of local anaesthetics based on weight are shown in **Table 3**.

Local anaesthetic drugs	**Local anaesthetic doses according to body weight (mg kg^{-1})**				**Duration of anaesthesia (mean)**
	<5 kg	**6–10 kg**	**11–20 kg**	**>20 kg**	
0.5% Bupivacaine/ levobupivacaine [9, 11, 53, 54, 59, 60]	0.3–1	0.4–0.5	0.3–0.4	0.3	65–90 min
0.5% Ropivacaine [9, 53, 56]	0.5–1	0.5	0.5	0.5	45–105 min
0.5% Tetracaine [9, 25, 55]	0.2–0.6	0.4–0.5	0.3–0.4	0.2–0.3	75–105 min

Table 3. Recommended local anaesthetic dosages for spinal anaesthesia in infants and children (Remodified from Kokki [8]).

6.3. Adjuncts to local anaesthetics in paediatric spinal anaesthesia

The relatively short duration of action and exceedingly variable characteristics between individuals (such as duration on anaesthetic, analgesic and motor block action) are among the major limitations of single-injection spinal anaesthesia.

The addition of different types of adjuvant modifies the onset time, efficacy and duration of spinal block. However, it should be noted that subarachnoidally injected drugs are in close communication with neural tissue. Therefore, potential neurotoxicity should be considered before injecting any additive drugs (such as preservatives and antioxidants) into the cerebrospinal fluid [11, 57]. The use of preservative-free additives seems to be a safe method that avoids these neurotoxic risks.

The fentanyl, clonidine and adrenaline are among the most commonly used adjuvants. Adrenalin is a vasoactive additive and can be combined with local anaesthetics to prolong the duration and intensity of block. One of the first researchers to use adrenalin was Tyrell Gray in 1909. Isobaric bupivacaine combined with adrenaline (2–5 μg kg^{-1} of body weight) prolongs the duration of analgesia by up to 50% [54].

A study by Fösel et al. found that 0.5% bupivacaine combined with 1:200,000 adrenaline prolonged the duration of analgesia from 50 to 95 min [58].

Opioids may also be used as adjunct. Low-dose intrathecal fentanyl (such as 0.2 μg kg^{-1} body weight) enhances the quality and extends the duration of spinal anaesthesia [59]. When used at high doses, fentanyl and morphine can give rise to a risk of delayed respiratory depression.

Clonidine is an alpha-2 agonist agent. Intra-spinal α2-adrenergic agonists induce analgesia by a pathway involving nitric oxide and acetylcholine release [60]. Cao et al. [61] found that 1 $\mu g\ kg^{-1}$ of body weight preservative-free clonidine combined with bupivacaine prolonged the duration of sensory and motor blocks by 30 min and postoperative analgesia by 120 min without affecting the hemodynamic stability.

7. Complications of spinal anaesthesia

Recent studies have shown that post-puncture complications in children are similar to those seen in adults after spinal anaesthesia [9]. However, evaluating the signs and symptoms of complications is more difficult in infants and young children compared with older children and adults. Babies can express their grievances with physiological changes and physical behaviours rather than verbally. Clinicians may misinterpret physical and behavioural changes as post-puncture complications.

Postdural complications and the incidence of severity are closely related to puncture technique. These complications include headache, backache, neurological complications, nausea and vomiting and cardiorespiratory and haemodynamic changes. More frequent complications are discussed below.

7.1. Headache

Headache is the most well-known complication of spinal anaesthesia [62].The incidence of headache was 3–4% with a 25–27 G spinal needle according to Kokki et al. [63]. A larger diameter needle (such as 22G) increases the incidence of post-puncture headache.

In order to decrease the risk of postdural puncture headache, small diameter atraumatic needles with a stylet were developed. These atraumatic needles are associated with a lower incidence and severity of puncture complications [64].

Indeed, headache is a common symptom in children after various surgical procedures, whatever the type of anaesthesia.

However, the symptoms mentioned below are mostly diagnostic of post-puncture headache:

- Postdural puncture headache is often bilateral.
- Develops within 24 h after lumbar puncture.
- Symptoms worsen in minutes by moving to a sitting position from their cumbent position.
- Some children may experience nausea and vomiting accompanied by symptoms such as blurred vision, vertigo and tinnitus [11].

These symptoms generally disappear spontaneously within 3–5 days, but in some children, they may continue for a few days.

Bed rest, hydration and the use of non-opioid analgesics and caffeine are mentioned in the treatment protocol.

An epidural blood patch may be required in prolonged cases and those not responding to treatment.

7.2. Backache

Backache is a common postoperative symptom. The incidence of backache after spinal anaesthesia is between 5% and 10% [9, 11, 41]. Backache may occur for various reasons such as direct trauma caused by the needle, ligamentous damage, muscular haematoma, reflex muscular spasm and uncomfortable positioning of the patient. Low back pain is the third most common pain in school-aged children. However, it is not known precisely what proportion of backache is associated with spinal anaesthesia.

7.3. Neurological complications

Looking at the overall epidemiology of neurological complications of spinal anaesthesia, they appear to be rare and transient. Improper patient selection, improper anaesthetic technique and inexperience may cause nerve damage, compressive haematoma and rarely definitive haematoma. However, these complications are rare.

The 1-year long, prospective ADARFEF study published by the French-Language Society of Paediatric Anaesthesiology in 1996 [65] evaluated complications of regional anaesthesia. Of 24,409 blocks, 60% were central blocks and 1.3% were spinal blocks. Most of the reported complications were minor (0.09%), emerged at the beginning of the process in the operating theatre, and had a short duration. Permanent neurological damage related to either spinal anaesthesia or other regional anaesthesia techniques has not been reported.

Some cases may develop transient neurological symptoms possibly because of subclinical neurotoxicity of local anaesthetic. Such symptoms occur a few hours after complete recovery from spinal anaesthesia. The incidence of symptoms following the use of bupivacaine has been reported as 3–4%. Symptoms are often mild and electropathological testing is negative [11].

Children may complain of pain radiating to lower extremities in the gluteal region and a tingling sensation in their feet. The intensity of pain ranges from mild to severe.

In recent years, ultrasound technology has offered new opportunities in the practice of regional anaesthesia, particularly in young children. Ultrasound guidance (USG) allows all relevant anatomical and neuroaxial structures to be visualised in infants up to 3 months old [66]. In experienced hands, USG may reduce the number of complications and improve the quality, safety and efficacy of neuraxial blocks in children. Therefore, the majority of paediatric anaesthesiologists are seeking to enhance their experiences in the use of USG in their routine clinical practice of paediatric spinal anaesthesia.

8. Summary

Paediatric spinal anaesthesia has made significant progress since Bier and Gray. Nevertheless, concerns about local anaesthetic toxicity, inexperience and the easy application of general anaesthesia except in high-risk conditions, causes do not favour the use of the paediatric spinal technique by an anaesthesiologist.

Continuous progress including developments in local anaesthetics with advanced training and appropriate use of drugs, paediatric equipment and ultrasound techniques have improved safety and efficacy in paediatric patients.

As anaesthesiologists become more experienced, paediatric spinal anaesthesia will continue to be an essential part of overall care not only for high-risk patients but also for patients undergoing elective surgery.

Author details

Esra Caliskan

Address all correspondence to: duru5654@gmail.com

Department of Anaesthesiology and Reanimation, Baskent University Faculty of Medicine, Ankara, Turkey

References

[1] Bier A. Versuche uber cocainisirung des ruckenmarkes (Experiments on the cocainization of the spinal cord). Deutsche Zeitschrift fur Chirurgie (in German) 1899; **51**: 361–369.

[2] Bier A, Donitz A. Munchener Medicinische Wochenschrift (Munich Weekly Medical) 1904; **51**: 593–596.

[3] Gray HT. A study of spinal anaesthesia in children and infants. Lancet 1909; Part I. 2: 913-917, Part II. 2: 991–996.

[4] Gray HT. A further study of spinal anaesthesia in children and infants. Lancet 1910; **1** (June 11): 1611–1616.

[5] Harnik EV, Hoy GR, Potolicchio S, Stewart DR, Siegalman RE. Spinal anesthesia in premature infants recovering from respiratory distress syndrome. Anesthesiology 1986; **64**: 95–99.

[6] Welborn LG, Rice LJ, Hannallah RS, Broadman LM, Ruttimann UE, Fink R. Postoperative apnoea in former preterm infants: prospective comparison of spinal and general anesthesia. Anesthesiology 1990; **72**: 838–842.

[7] Krane EJ, Haberkern CM, Jacobson LE. Postoperative apnea, bradycardia, and oxygen desaturation in formerly premature infants: prospective comparison of spinal and general anesthesia. Anesth Analg 1995; **80**: 7–13.

[8] Somri M, Gaitini L, Vaida S, Collins G, Sabo E, Mogilner G. Postoperative outcome in high-risk infants undergoing herniorrhaphy: comparison between spinal and general anaesthesia. Anaesthesia 1998; **53**: 762–766.

[9] Kokki H. Spinal blocks. Paediatr Anaesth 2012; **22**: 56–64. DOI:10.111/j.1460-9592.2011.03693

[10] Sahin F, Selcuki M, Ecin N et al. Level of conus medullaris in term and preterm neonates. Arch Dis Child Fetal Neonatal Ed 1997; **77**: F67–F69.

[11] Kokki H. Spinal anaesthesia in infants and children. Best Pract Clin Res Anaesthesiol 2000; **14**: 687–707. DOI: 10.1053/bean.2000.0121

[12] Gupta A, Saha U. Spinal anesthesia in children: a review. J Anaesthesiol Clin Pharmacol 2014; **30**: 10–18. DOI: 10.4103/0970-9185.125687

[13] Frawley G, Ingelmo P. Spinal anaesthesia in the neonate. Best Pract Res Clin Anaesthesiol 2010; **24**: 337–351.

[14] Shin SK, Hong JY, Kim WO, Koo BN, Kim JE, Kil HK. Ultrasound evaluation of the sacral area and comparison of sacral interspinous and hiatal approach for caudal block in children. Anesthesiology 2009; **111**: 1135–1140. DOI: 10.1097/ALN.0b013e3181bc6dd4

[15] Shenkman Z, Rathaus V, Jedeikin R et al. The distance from the skin to the subarachnoid space can be predicted in premature infants. Can J Anaesth 2004; **51(2)**: 160–162.

[16] Ecoffey C, Dubousset AM, Samii K. Lumbar and thoracic epidural anesthesia for urologic and upper abdominal surgery in infants and children. Anesth Analg 1986; **65**: 87–90.

[17] Porter RW, Hibbert C, Wellmann P. Backache and the lumbar spinal canal. Spine Spine (Phila Pa 1976) 1980; **5**: 99–105.

[18] Lee SJ, Ralston HJ, Drey EA, Partridge JC, Rosen MA. Fetal pain: a systematic multidisciplinary review of the evidence. JAMA 2005; **294**: 947–954. DOI: 10.1001/jama.294.8.947

[19] Oberlander TF, Berde CB, Lam KH, Rappaport LA, Saul JP. Infants tolerate spinal anesthesia with minimal overall autonomic changes: analysis of heart rate variability in former premature infants undergoing hernia repair. Anesth Analg 1995; **80(1)**: 20–27.

[20] Jevtovic-Todorovic V, Absalom AR, Blomgren K, et al. Anaesthetic neurotoxicity and neuroplasticity: an expert group report and statement based on the BJA Salzburg Seminar. Br J Anaesth 2013; **111**: 143–151. DOI: 10.1093/bja/aet177

[21] Istaphanous GK, Ward CG, Nan X, et al. Characterization and quantification of isoflurane-induced developmental apoptotic cell death in mouse cerebral cortex. Anesth Analg 2013; **116**: 845–854. DOI: 10.1213/ANE.0b013e318281e988

[22] Sanders RD, Davidson A. Anesthetic induced neurotoxicity of the neonate: time for clinical guidelines? Pediatric Anesth 2009; **19**: 1141–1146. DOI: 10.1111/J.1460-9592.2009.03141

[23] Davidson AJ, Disma N, de Graaff JC et al. Neurodevelopmental outcome at 2 years of age after general anaesthesia and awake-regional anaesthesia in infancy (GAS): an international multicentre, randomised controlled trial. Lancet 2016; **387**: 239–250. DOI: 10.1016/S0140-6736(15)00608-X

[24] Takasaki M. Ventilation and ventilatory response to carbon dioxide during caudal anaesthesia with lidocaine or bupivacaine in sedated children. Acta Anaesthesiol Scand 1988; **32**: 218–221.

[25] Williams RK, Adams DC, Aladjem EV et al. The safety and efficacy of spinal anesthesia for surgery in infants: Vermont Infant Spinal Registry. Anesth Analg 2006; **102**: 67–71. DOI: 10.1213/01.ANE.0000159162.86033.21

[26] Bosenberg A. Benefits of regional anesthesia in children. Paediatr Anesth 2012; **22**: 10–18. DOI: 10.1111/j.1460-9592.2011.03691.x

[27] Zwass M, Gregory GA. Pediatric and neonatal intensive care. In: Miller RD, editor. Miller's Anesthesia. 7th ed. Philadelphia: Churchill Livingstone Elsevier; 2010. pp. 2654–2703.

[28] Williams RK, Abajian JC. High spinal anesthesia for repair of patent ductus arteriosus in neonates. Paediatr Anesth 1997; **7**: 205–209.

[29] Polaner DM, Drescher J. Pediatric regional anesthesia: what is the current safety record? Paediatr Anesth 2011; **21**: 737–742. DOI: 10.1111/j.1460-9592.2010.03499.x

[30] Burton D, Nicholson G, Hall G. Endocrine and metabolic response to surgery. Contin Educ Anaesth Crit Care Pain 2004; **4**: 144–147. DOI: 10.1093/bjaceaccp/mkh040

[31] Russell P, von Ungern-Sternberg BS, Schug SA. Perioperative analgesia in pediatric surgery. Curr Opin Anaesthesiol 2013; **26**: 420–427. DOI: 10.1097/ACO.0b013e3283625cc8

[32] Bosenberg A. Paediatric regional anaesthesia update. Paediatr Anaesth 2004; **14**: 398–402. DOI: 10.1111/j.1460-9592.2004.01338.x

[33] Bozkurt P. The analgesic efficacy and neuroendocrine response in paediatric patients treated with two analgesic techniques: using morphine-epidural and patient-controlled analgesia. Paediatr Anaesth 2002; **12**: 248–254.

[34] Wolf AR, Doyle E, Thomas E. Modifying infant stress responses to major surgery: spinal vs extradural vs opioid analgesia. Paediatr Anaesth 1998; **8**: 305–311.

[35] Wolf AR. Effects of regional analgesia on stress responses to pediatric surgery. Paediatr Anesth 2012; **22**: 19–24. DOI: 10.1111/j.1460-9592.2011.03714.x

[36] Cassady JF Jr, Lederhaas G, Cancel DD, Cummings RJ, Loveless EA. A randomized comparison of the effects of continuous thoracic epidural analgesia and intravenous patient-controlled analgesia after posterior spinal fusion in adolescents. Reg Anesth Pain Med 2000; **25**: 246–253.

[37] Dalens B. Regional anesthesia in children. Anesth Analg 1989; **68**: 654–672.

[38] Abajian JC, Mellish RW, Browne AF, Perkins FM, Lambert DH, Mazuzan JE Jr. Spinal anesthesia for surgery in the high risk infant. Anesth Analg 1984; **63**: 359–362.

[39] Holzman RS. Airway management. In: Davis PJ, Cladis FP, Motoyoma EK editors. Smith's Anesthesia for Infants and Children. 8th ed. Philadelphia: Elsevier Mosby; 2011. pp. 344–364 ISBN: 978-0-323-06612-9.

[40] Smith AH, Gay JC, Patel NR. Trends in resource utilization associated with the inpatient treatment of neonatal congenital heart disease. Congenit Heart Dis 2014; **9**: 96–105. DOI: 10.1111/chd.12103

[41] Kachko L, Birk E, Simhi E, Tzeitlin E, Freud E, Katz J. Spinal anesthesia for noncardiac surgery in infants with congenital heart diseases. Pediatr Anaesth 2012; **22**: 647–653.

[42] White MC. Approach to managing children with heart disease for noncardiac surgery. Paediatr Anesth 2011; **21**: 522–529. DOI: 10.1111/j.1460-9592.2010.03416.x

[43] Kokki H. Spinal Anesthesia in Children–Evaluation of Puncture Characteristics of Various Needles and Block Efficacy of Various Local Anesthetic Solutions. Kuopio: Koupio University Printing Office 2000.

[44] Faillace WJ, Warrier I, Canady AI. Paraplegia after lumbar puncture. In an infant with previously undiagnosed hemophilia A. Treatment and perioperative considerations. Clin Pediatr (Phila) 1989; **28**: 136–138.

[45] Gleason CA, Martin RJ, Anderson JV, Carlo WA, Sanniti KJ, Fanaroff AA. Optimal position for a spinal tap in preterm infants. Pediatrics 1983; **71**: 31–35.

[46] Kokki H, Hendolin H. Comparison of 25 G and 29 G Quincke spinal needles in paediatric day case surgery. A prospective randomized study of the puncture characteristics, success rate and postoperative complaints. Paediatr Anaesth 1996; **6**: 115–119. DOI: 10.1111/j.1460-9592.1996.tb00372.x

[47] Apiliogullari S, Duman A, Gok F, Akillioglu I. Spinal needle design and size affect the incidence of postdural puncture headache in children. Paediatr Anaesth 2010; **20**: 177–182. DOI: 10.1111/j.1460-9592.2009.03236.x

[48] Rice LJ, DeMars PD, Whalen TV, Crooms JC, Parkinson SK. Duration of spinal anesthesia in infants less than one year of age. Comparison of three hyperbaric techniques. Reg Anesth 1994; **19**: 325–329.

[49] Sale SM. Neonatal apnoea. Best Pract Res Clin Anaesthesiol 2010; **24**: 323–336.

[50] Vilo S, Rautiainen P, Kaisti K et al. Pharmacokinetics of intravenous dexmedetomidine in children under 11 yr of age. Br J Anaesth 2008; **100**: 697–700. DOI: 10.1093/bja/aen070

[51] Ross AK, Bryskin RB. Regional anesthesia. In: Davis PJ, Cladis FP, Motoyoma EK editors. Smith's Anesthesia for Infants and Children. 8th ed. Philadelphia: Elsevier Mosby; 2011. pp. 452–458. ISBN: 978-0-323-06612-9.

[52] Berde CB, Strichartz GR. Local anesthetics. In: Miller RD, editor. Miller's Anesthesia. 7th ed. Philadelphia: Churchill Livingstone Elsevier; 2010. pp. 913–939. ISBN: 978-0-443-06959-8.ch30.

[53] Frawley G, Smith KR, Ingelmo P. Relative potencies of bupivacaine, levobupivacaine, and ropivacaine for neonatal spinal anaesthesia. Br J Anaesth 2009; **103**: 731–738. DOI: 10.1093/bja/aep259

[54] MaheV, Ecoffey C. Spinal anesthesia with isobaric bupivacaine in infants. Anesthesiology 1988; **68**: 601–603.

[55] Kokki H, Tuovinen K, Hendolin H. Spinal anaesthesia for paediatric day-case surgery: a double-blind, randomized, parallel group, prospective comparison of isobaric and hyperbaric bupivacaine. Br J Anaesth 1998; **81**: 502–506. DOI: 10.1093/bja/81.4.502

[56] Kokki H, Ylönen P, Laisalmi M et al. Isobaric ropivacaine 5 mg/ml for spinal anesthesia in children. Anesth Analg 2005; **100**: 66–70.

[57] Walker SM, Yaksh TL. Neuraxial analgesia in neonates and infants: a review of clinical and preclinical strategies for the development of safety and efficacy data. Anesth Analg 2012; **115**: 638–662. DOI: 10.1213/ANE.0b013e31826253f2

[58] Fösel T, Wilhelm W, Grüness V, Molter G. Spinal anesthesia in infancy using bupivacaine 0.5%. The effect of an adrenaline addition on duration and hemodynamics. Anaesthetist 1994; **43**: 26–29.

[59] Batra YK, Locesh VC, Panda NB et al. Dose-response study of intrathecal fentanyl added to bupivacaine in infants undergoing lower abdominal and urologic surgery. Paediatr Anesth 2008; **18**: 613–616. DOI: 10.1111/j.1460-9592.2008.02613.x

[60] Rochette A, Raux O, Troncin R, Dadure C, Verdier R, Capdevila X. Clonidine prolongs spinal anesthesia in newborns: a prospective dose-ranging study. Anesth Analg 2004; **98**: 56–59. DOI: 10.1213/01.ANE.0000093229.17729.6C

[61] Cao JP, Miao XY, Liu J, Shi XY. An evaluation of intrathecal bupivacaine combined with intrathecal or intravenous clonidine in children undergoing orthopedic surgery: a randomized double-blinded study. Paediatr Anaesth 2011; **21**: 399–405. DOI: 10.1111/j.1460-9592.2011.03543.x

[62] Janssens E, Aerssens P, Alliët P, Gillis P, Raes M. Postdural puncture headaches in children. A literature review. Eur J Pediatr 2003; **162**: 117–121. DOI: 10.1007/s00431-002-1122-6

[63] Kokki H, Salonvaara M, Herrgård E, Onen P. Postdural puncture headache is not an age-related symptom in children: a prospective, open randomized, parallel group study comparing a 22-gauge Quincke with a 22-Gauge Whitacre needle. Paediatr Anesth 1999; **9**: 429–434. DOI: 10.1046/j.1460-9592.1999.00398.x

[64] Kokki H, Turunen M, Heikkinen M, Reinikainen M, Laisalmi M. High success rate and low incidence of headache and neurological symptoms with two spinal needle designs in children. Acta Anaesthesiol Scand 2005; **49**: 1367–1372. DOI: 10.1111/j.1399-6576.2005.00837.x

[65] Ecoffey C, Lacroix F, Giaufré E, Orliaguet G, Courrèges P; Association des Anesthésistes Réanimateurs Pédiatriques d'Expression Française (ADARPEF). Epidemiology and morbidity of regional anesthesia in children: a follow-up one-year prospective survey of the French-Language Society of Paediatric Anaesthesiologists (ADARPEF). Paediatr Anaesth 2010; **20**: 1061–1069. DOI: 10.1111/j.1460-9592.2010.03448

[66] Rubin K, Sullivan D, Sadhasivam S. Are peripheral and neuraxial blocks with ultrasound guidance more effective and safe in children? Paediatr Anaesth 2009; **19**: 92–96. DOI: 10.1111/j.1460-9592.2008.02918

Section 3

Diagnosis and Management of Neonatal Tumors

Chapter 4

Neonatal Tumors

Kenneth W. Gow and Matthew Dellinger

Additional information is available at the end of the chapter

http://dx.doi.org/10.5772/68070

Abstract

Neonatal tumors encompass a group of heterogeneous neoplasms that demonstrate anatomic locations, behavior patterns, histologic features, and treatment responses that are distinct from neoplasms found in older children. The majority of neonatal tumors are benign, with malignant lesions accounting for only 2% of childhood cancers. However, histologically benign tumors can lead to detrimental effects on the fetus and newborn due to their size and location in relation to vital structures. An understanding of the incidence, appearance, and typical locations of neonatal tumors can provide important diagnostic information and guide treatment decisions. Although surgical intervention is the mainstay of therapy for many neonatal tumors, it is important to recognize that some lesions will regress spontaneously, whereas others may respond to noninvasive treatment modalities. In this chapter, we explore the epidemiology of neonatal tumors and provide a location-based classification schema to aid in diagnosis. A summary of the presentation, diagnosis, and management of the most common neonatal tumors is provided as well.

Keywords: neonatal tumors, sacrococcygeal teratoma, neuroblastoma, infantile hepatic hemangioma, mesenchymal hamartoma, ovarian cyst, cervical lymphatic malformation, rhabdomyosarcoma, congenital mesoblastic nephroma

1. Introduction

Neonatal tumors encompass a group of heterogeneous neoplasms that are diagnosed prenatally or within the first 30 days of life. Neonatal tumors demonstrate anatomic locations, behavior patterns, histologic features, and treatment responses that are distinct from neoplasms found in older children [1]. The preponderance of information regarding the epidemiology of neonatal tumors is provided through the experience of single institutions. The true incidence of these lesions is unknown, as studies do not always account for pregnancies with a prenatally diagnosed mass that end in stillbirth, miscarriage, or early termination of pregnancy.

Most solid neoplasms identified in neonates are benign [2]. The incidence of a malignant tumor is 1 in every 12,500–27,500 live births, accounting for 2% of all childhood cancers [1]. Distinguishing between benign and malignant neoplasms can prove to be challenging in this group of patients. The features of a tumor that denote malignancy in adults, such as high nuclear-cytoplasmic ratio, high mitotic rate, and anaplasia, may be present in benign lesions in children and neonates [3]. Neonatal tumors are also unique in that they arise from embryonic and immature tissue as a result of intrinsic dysfunction of cellular growth and proliferation [3, 4]. As opposed to adult tumors, environmental exposures are believed to play little to no role in tumorigenesis [4]. Some malignant lesions have minimal potential for invasion or metastasis, while histologically benign lesions can be lethal due to their size and location.

Although less than 10% of childhood cancers arise in the setting of a cancer predisposition syndrome, any neonatal tumor should raise concern for this possibility [5]. The presence of associated congenital anomalies, multifocal or bilateral disease, and cancer in close relatives is suggestive of an underlying cancer predisposition syndrome [6]. Several specific types of tumors, including retinoblastoma, adrenocortical carcinoma, pleuropulmonary blastoma, hepatoblastoma, and Wilms' tumor, show a strong association with a cancer predisposition syndrome [5]. Since the presence of genetically derived lesions can have implications for these children and their family members, genetic counseling and testing should be offered.

2. Diagnosis

A thorough history and physical examination are paramount in the evaluation of a newborn. However, many anomalies can be detected prior to birth. The ability to diagnose neoplasms in utero has evolved significantly with improvement in imaging modalities. Fetal ultrasonography, magnetic resonance imaging (MRI), and echocardiography offer physicians the opportunity to diagnose a variety of congenital diseases in the prenatal period [7–9]. Ultrasonography is a critical component of the prenatal obstetric evaluation and is currently the standard of care. Prenatal ultrasound provides vital information regarding gestational age, number of fetuses, fetal health, and the presence of congenital anomalies [9]. Ultrasound and MRI are preferred because they avoid the damaging effects of ionizing radiation.

For decades, ultrasonography has been the principal imaging modality for prenatal diagnosis of fetal anomalies [10]. The benefits of ultrasound are numerous, including wide availability, low cost, noninvasiveness, and the ability, to provide real-time evaluation of the fetus. One shortcoming of ultrasound is that results are operator dependent and can vary with the experience and expertise of the examiner [11]. In a systematic review of ultrasound for fetal assessment in early pregnancy, Bricker et al. [12] determined the overall sensitivity for detection of fetal anomalies to be 44.7%. However, the sensitivities of the included studies showed great variability, ranging from 15 to 85.3%. In addition to operator experience, gestational age, anomaly type, and equipment quality impact the accuracy of screening prenatal ultrasound [12].

In the past two decades, magnetic resonance imaging (MRI) has become increasingly utilized as an adjunct to ultrasound in the evaluation of fetal and neonatal anomalies [8, 10, 13].

http://dx.doi.org/10.5772/68070

One driving force behind this phenomenon is the development of ultrafast MRI, which limits fetal motion artifact and does not require maternal-fetal sedation [11]. The greatest utility of MRI appears to occur in cases where sonographic findings are equivocal or further diagnostic information is desired [11, 14, 15]. MRI is also particularly useful in illustrating anatomic relationships between neoplasms and adjacent structures, characterizing intracranial and soft tissue lesions, in cases of oligohydramnios and in cases of maternal obesity [11, 14, 15].

In the most recent Guidelines for Diagnostic Imaging in Pregnancy and Lactation, the American College of Obstetricians and Gynecologists states that there is no evidence of harm from tissue heating, acoustic damage, or teratogenesis when using MRI in pregnancy [16]. However, one issue that merits discussion is the use of gadolinium contrast dye to enhance fetal imaging. In practice, gadolinium is administered as a gadolinium-chelate molecule that is water-soluble and can cross the placenta into fetal circulation. Following filtration and excretion by the fetal kidneys, these molecules can accumulate in amniotic fluid with the ability to release potentially toxic gadolinium ions [17]. Although the effect of free gadolinium ions on the fetus is unknown, the current recommendation is to abstain from the routine use of MRI contrast agents unless the benefits can be shown to clearly outweigh this theoretical risk [17].

The diagnosis of a neonatal tumor has a profound emotional impact on a family and raises questions about accuracy of diagnosis, prognosis, treatment options, and long-term outcomes [18]. While technological improvements in imaging modalities have led to better sensitivity in diagnosing congenital anomalies, the false-positive rate is far from negligible [19]. Care should be taken in making definitive statements about diagnosis and prognosis on prenatal imaging as normal anatomic variants can have the appearance of a neoplastic process and some lesions will regress spontaneously. Conversely, sonographic findings of polyhydramnios, fetal hydrops, hepatosplenomegaly, and placentomegaly should raise suspicion for an undiagnosed tumor.

Finally, having diagnostic imaging that points to anomalies will allow the care team to have prenatal discussions and do important planning. Depending on all tests done, the parents should be offered possible diagnoses, complications, and outcomes. However, one needs to be guarded with prognostication, and consideration for termination of the pregnancy must be very carefully made including all knowns and unknowns. Assuming that the plans are for delivery, early diagnosis will allow for planning around the delivery; the location of the birthing center (closer to home vs. in a maternal-neonatal center), the means of birth (vaginal vs. Cesarean section vs. ex utero intrapartum treatment (EXIT)), the personnel required for the birth aside from those needed to care for the mother (neonatologist, pediatric anesthesiologist, pediatric otolaryngologist, pediatric general surgeon, pediatric cardiothoracic surgeon), and logistics with regard to coordination of the team including diagnostic and operative services.

3. Anatomic considerations/locations

Neonatal tumors represent a varied group of neoplasms that are discovered in multiple locations throughout the body (**Figure 1**). The diversity observed is not surprising since these lesions arise

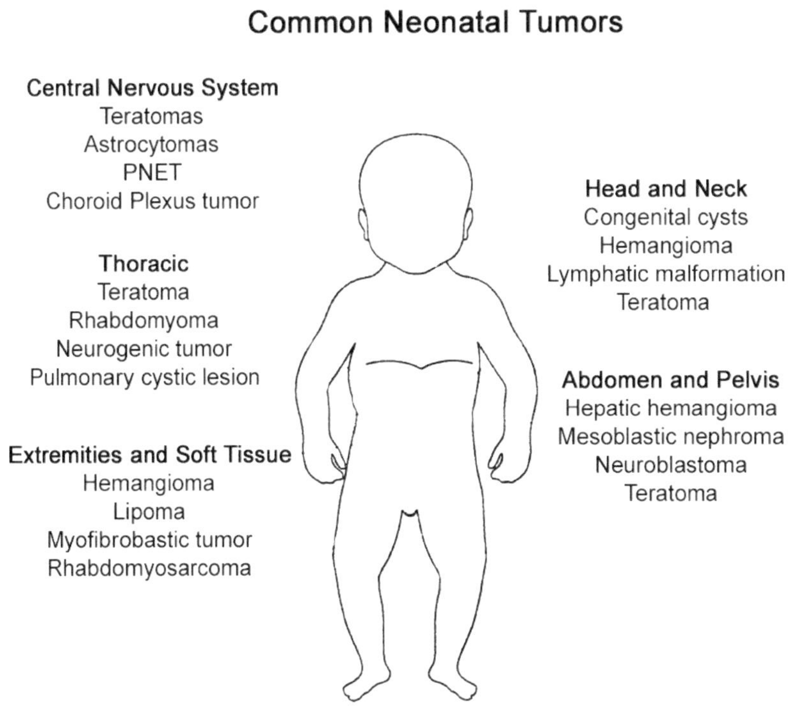

Figure 1. Common neonatal tumors based on location.

from abnormalities in fetal and neonatal development. Teratomas, particularly sacrococcygeal teratomas, are the most common neonatal tumor [1, 20, 21]. Neuroblastoma is the second most common neoplasm in neonates and the leading cause of malignancy in this group of patients. In order to decrease frequency, soft tissue tumors, central nervous system (CNS) tumors, leukemia, and renal tumors are the next most common tumor types recognized [1, 20, 21]. **Table 1** provides a brief summary of the most frequently encountered neonatal tumors. Knowledge of the incidence, appearance, and typical locations of these lesions can provide important diagnostic

Type	Percentage
Extracranial teratoma	24–30%
Neuroblastoma	23–30%
Soft tissue tumors	8–12%
Leukemia	6–12%
CNS tumors	6–10%
Renal tumors	5–7%
Hepatic tumors	5%
Cardiopulmonary tumors	<3%

Table 1. Distribution of commonly occurring neonatal tumors [1, 18, 20, 21].

http://dx.doi.org/10.5772/68070

information. In particular, the location of the lesion gives a wealth of information regarding the differential diagnosis. The following discussions provide a location-based review of common neonatal tumors, which is intended to provide the clinician a basis to create a differential diagnosis to plan for management. Later, specific histologic diseases will be presented to allow tailoring of therapy.

4. Central nervous system

Primary central nervous system (CNS) neoplasms are the most common solid tumor in childhood and the leading cause of cancer death in this group of patients [22]. Fortunately, this is a rare entity with an estimated incidence of 5.57 cases per 100,000 children between the ages of 0 and 19 [23]. In neonates, CNS tumors are the fifth most common solid malignancy, which occur less frequently than lesions found in older children. Brain tumors in fetuses and neonates are unique in that they are often supratentorial, while lesions in older children are typically infratentorial [24]. The rarity of neonatal brain tumors and the absence of a national pediatric CNS cancer registry make it difficult to ascertain a true incidence [25].

In a retrospective review of 250 cases of perinatal brain tumors, Isaacs [24] found that the most common tumors were teratomas (29.6%), astrocytomas (18.8%), primitive neuroectodermal tumors (13.2%), and choroid plexus tumors (13.2%). Those children presenting with choroid plexus tumors, low-grade astrocytomas, and gangliogliomas had the best survival, while intracranial teratomas and neuroectodermal tumors exhibited the worst prognosis [24]. The 5-year survival rate for neonatal brain tumors, regardless of treatment modality, is 23–36% [25]. The management of these patients includes surgical resection, chemotherapy, and irradiation, although any treatment decision should be coordinated through a multidisciplinary approach. Regardless of the histologic subtype and associated prognosis, the identification of a neonatal brain tumor is a devastating and life-altering experience for families.

5. Head and neck

Multiple conditions lead to the development of masses occurring in the head and neck of pediatric patients. The differential diagnosis is extensive and includes a variety of congenital, inflammatory, benign, and malignant lesions [26]. The vast majority of these lesions are benign. According to a comprehensive, 5-year review of 445 pediatric neck masses at Children's Hospital of Philadelphia, the most frequent lesions were congenital in origin (55%), followed by inflammatory masses (27%), malignant neoplasms (11%), and benign neoplasms (3%) [27]. Inflammatory lesions likely account for the most common pediatric neck masses but often resolve with conservative therapy, obviating the need for biopsy or excision [26]. The incidence and distribution of head and neck masses in the neonatal period are not as well defined.

The most common congenital head and neck lesions are branchial cleft, thyroglossal duct, and dermoid cysts. Although less common, vascular masses, lymphatic malformations, and teratomas deserve special consideration secondary to the potential to cause detrimental effects on the developing fetus and newborn. Highly vascular lesions can lead to high-output cardiac failure and hydrops fetalis. Fluid accumulation in lymphatic malformations and the nearby tissues can also lead to fetal hydrops. Mass effect and extrinsic compression from certain lesions have the potential to cause life-threatening airway obstruction as well as atypical development of adjacent structures. Cervical lymphatic malformations and cervical teratomas, two lesions responsible for these physiologic disturbances, will be discussed in greater detail later in this chapter.

Cervical vascular masses include congenital and infantile hemangiomas. An important distinction to make is that vascular malformations and congenital hemangiomas are present at birth, grow concurrently with the child, and do not involute. Vascular tumors develop in the neonatal period and demonstrate a proliferative phase followed by involution [28]. Infantile hemangiomas occur in up to 4–5% of newborns [29]. Infantile hemangiomas arise following birth, proliferate for a variable amount of time, and ultimately involute. In contrast, congenital hemangiomas proliferate in utero and are fully developed at birth. These masses can be subdivided into rapidly involuting and noninvoluting types. Congenital hemangiomas are rare, accounting for only 3% of all hemangiomas [30].

Malignant head and neck lesions are rarely diagnosed in neonates. Lymphomas are the most common head and neck malignancy in children, with 60% of these tumors being classified as non-Hodgkin's lymphoma and the remaining 40% classified as Hodgkin's lymphoma [31]. Excisional biopsy is usually necessary to provide adequate tissue to confirm the diagnosis. Following diagnosis, a multidisciplinary approach is recommended for appropriate staging and treatment [31]. Neuroblastoma is another malignancy that can be found in the head and neck of neonates. Typically, these are metastatic lesions as primary cervical neuroblastoma accounts for only 5% of neonatal neuroblastoma [32]. Some children may have a concomitant Horner's syndrome secondary to compression of the cervical sympathetic chain. Treatment of neuroblastoma is also conducted via a multidisciplinary approach, with lesions diagnosed prenatally having a better prognosis than those identified following birth [32]. Other neonatal head and neck cancers include salivary gland malignancies, thyroid cancer, and nasopharyngeal carcinoma, each of which is exceedingly rare in this population.

6. Thoracic

The differential diagnosis of fetal and neonatal thoracic tumors can be narrowed significantly with an understanding of their incidence and common locations. One useful method for organizing these tumors is to differentiate between mediastinal, pleural, and pulmonary neoplasms.

The anterior mediastinum includes the region between the sternum and pericardium below the thoracic inlet. The thymus, portions of the thyroid gland, and nodal tissue serve as potential sites for tumorigenesis. In a retrospective review of 534 fetuses and neonates diagnosed with teratomas, Isaacs [33] found that 2.6% of these masses occurred in the mediastinum. Teratomas that do occur in this region are usually located in the anterior mediastinum [34]. Sonographic identification of calcifications can help differentiate mediastinal teratomas from congenital pulmonary airway malformations and pulmonary sequestration [35]. Large mediastinal teratomas have the potential to cause lethal sequelae for the fetus and newborn. Polyhydramnios and preterm labor may develop from esophageal obstruction. High-output cardiac failure secondary to solid lesions with high vascularity can lead to fetal hydrops and intrauterine death. Perinatal decompensation and death are risks associated with intrathoracic airway obstruction. Although the thymus is included in the anterior mediastinum, thymomas are exceptionally rare in children, with most of the published cases being limited to case reports and retrospective reviews. Thyroid neoplasms and lymphoma are also extremely rare in this group of patients.

The middle mediastinum encompasses the heart and pericardium, great vessels, tracheal bifurcation, and phrenic nerves. Primary cardiac tumors are very uncommon in the fetus and neonate [36]. Of the primary cardiac tumors that occur in these patients, nearly all of them are histologically benign [37, 38]. Rhabdomyomas account for the majority of these lesions [36–38]. Fibromas, myxomas, and teratomas represent additional benign cardiac lesions with rare occurrence. Pericardial-based teratomas are also exceedingly rare. Based on their size and location, middle mediastinal tumors can have a number of detrimental physiologic effects. Dysrhythmias, impairment of cardiac function, and great vessel compression may result in fetal or neonatal demise without timely intervention.

The posterior mediastinum is bound by the pericardium and thoracic vertebrae and extends from the sternal notch inferiorly to the diaphragm. The esophagus, descending thoracic aorta, azygos veins, thoracic duct, and neural tissue are the key components of this region. Nearly all of the tumors arising in the posterior mediastinum in children are neurogenic in origin. Neurogenic tumors are named according to the type of neural tissue from which they originate. Neoplasms that arise from the sympathetic chain reflect a continuum of cellular differentiation and maturation [39]. Ganglioneuromas are benign, fully differentiated, and arise from mature Schwann and ganglion cells. These are the most common posterior mediastinal masses in children [39]. Ganglioneuroblastomas are malignant tumors of intermediate differentiation and contain both mature and immature elements of ganglion cells [39]. Neuroblastomas are also malignant tumors that are derived from immature, undifferentiated ganglion cells [39]. Neuroblastoma is the most common malignancy and second most common tumor in neonates, with approximately 5% arising in the posterior mediastinum [32]. Additional tumors include neurofibroma, neurilemoma, neurosarcoma, and paraganglioma, all of which are uncommon in neonates.

Pulmonary lesions diagnosed prenatally or in the newborn are rarely true neoplasms. The most commonly identified abnormalities are congenital pulmonary malformations, intra- and extralobar pulmonary sequestrations, and congenital lobar emphysema. Pleuropulmonary blastoma is a very rare, aggressive pulmonary malignancy. Although uncommon, it is the primary pulmonary malignancy presenting in childhood with up to 94% of cases being diagnosed in children 6 years of age and younger [40]. Type I and II pleuropulmonary blastomas possess cystic components, which can lead to misdiagnosis as benign lesions. Since pleuropulmonary blastoma is rare and over 90% of pulmonary cystic lesions in children are benign, surveillance may be an appropriate strategy with the knowledge that the emergence of solid components in the lesion warrants surgical resection [40].

7. Abdominal/retroperitoneal/pelvic

Masses discovered in the neonatal abdominal cavity, retroperitoneum, and pelvis represent a very diverse group of pathologies as would be expected based on the tissue types and organs in this region. These lesions range from small incidentally discovered masses to those occupying an entire body cavity, from benign to malignant and from purely cystic to solid neoplasms [41]. Hepatic lesions are the most common intra-abdominal neonatal tumors, while neuroblastoma and teratoma are the most common retroperitoneal and pelvic masses, respectively.

Hepatic tumors encompass a variety of benign and malignant lesions, representing only 5% of neonatal tumors. Most neonatal liver tumors are benign and discovered as an asymptomatic abdominal mass or identified on prenatal imaging [5]. In a retrospective review of 194 cases of fetal and neonatal hepatic tumors, Isaacs [42] identified hemangioma (60.3%), mesenchymal hamartoma (23.2%), and hepatoblastoma (16.5%) as the three primary tumor types. Hepatoblastoma represents the most common primary hepatic malignancy in this patient population. Serum alpha-fetoprotein is elevated in nearly half of neonates with hepatoblastoma; however, serum levels may remain elevated for several months following birth in children with benign hepatic masses or in the absence of hepatic masses [43]. Surgical resection is the primary treatment modality for hepatoblastoma with chemotherapy typically reserved for children with unresectable lesions or metastatic disease. Newborns presenting with congenital hepatoblastoma appear to have similar survival when compared to older children with similar stages of disease [43].

Renal tumors account for approximately 5–7% of neonatal tumors. Non-neoplastic pathologies, such as hydronephrosis and renal cystic disease, are far more prevalent than true neoplasms, accounting for up to 40% of neonatal abdominal masses [44]. The most common neonatal renal neoplasm is congenital mesoblastic nephroma (CMN), followed in frequency by Wilms' tumor, rhabdoid tumor, and clear cell sarcoma [44]. Juxtarenal masses are also part of the differential diagnosis with neuroblastoma being the most common of these lesions.

Although prenatal ultrasound is widely used, it is estimated that only 15% of renal masses are diagnosed prenatally [45]. Of those lesions not diagnosed via fetal ultrasound, nearly 50% are identified during routine physical examination [45]. Mesoblastic nephroma is rarely diagnosed following the first 3 months of life, while it is uncommon for Wilms' tumor to be diagnosed prior to 6 months of age [41]. Mesoblastic nephroma may be differentiated from other masses by the presence of a "ring sign" or anechoic circle surrounding the mass on sonography [46]. The optimal treatment for neonatal renal masses is surgical resection. Similar to hepatic lesions, chemotherapy is reserved for malignant lesions that are unresectable or metastatic at the time of diagnosis.

Teratomas are the most common neonatal tumors and the most prevalent pelvic neoplasms. In contrast, neonatal testicular tumors are rarely encountered in clinical practice. The tumors that do occur are usually testicular germ cell tumors such as teratomas and yolk sac tumors [47]. Diagnosis typically occurs after parents or clinicians palpate a testicular mass. Ultrasound examination distinguishes between intra- and extratesticular pathology. Yolk sac tumors are

http://dx.doi.org/10.5772/68070

the most common testicular malignancy in children, although most masses are benign. Serum alpha-fetoprotein (AFP) is a useful adjunct in the diagnosis of testicular tumors as it is elaborated by nearly 90% of yolk sac tumors in childhood [48]. However, measuring AFP levels is less reliable in newborns as they can physiologically remain elevated for up to 1 year after birth in the absence of underlying pathology. Since most of these lesions are benign, some tumors can be excised with a testicle-sparing approach [49]. In the event that a malignancy is identified on intraoperative frozen section, radical orchiectomy is required.

Ovarian enlargement can result from a variety of pathologies including ovarian cysts, ovarian torsion, and benign and malignant neoplasms [50]. Fortunately, true neonatal ovarian masses are infrequently seen in practice. Many lesions are identified on prenatal imaging, although some children present with palpable abdominal or groin masses, endocrine abnormalities, or ambiguous genitalia and congenital anomalies [50]. The majority of fetal and neonatal ovarian masses are cystic in nature. Management of ovarian cysts includes observation for simple lesions and surgical excision for larger, more complex lesions [41]. Preservation of functional ovarian parenchyma is the foundation of management.

8. Extremities and soft tissue

Soft tissue tumors comprise a heterogeneous group of benign and malignant neoplasms that represent 8–12% of neonatal tumors [1, 20, 21]. Soft tissue tumors are a rare entity in neonates, and the true incidence is unknown. There are a wide variety of benign tumors, including vascular malformations, lipomas, lipoblastomas, and fibroblastic tumors.

Head and neck hemangiomas are the most common benign soft tissue tumors in neonates. Lipomas consist of a group of widely distributed fatty tumors that are composed of mature adipocytes with a histologic appearance identical to normal fat [51]. Lipomas are classified based on their depth, with superficial lesions being much more common than deep lesions, which are located beneath the superficial fascia [51]. Lipoblastomas are rare, benign, rapidly growing tumors that arise from embryonic white fat and typically occur on the trunk and limbs [52]. The treatment of lipomas and lipoblastomas is usually complete excision, although the extent of resection should take functional and cosmetic outcomes into consideration. Fibroblastic and myofibroblastic tumors of intermediate prognosis represent benign lesions that display locally aggressive behavior with little to no propensity to metastasize [53]. Surgical resection remains the mainstay of treatment, yet a multidisciplinary approach is often necessary as radical resection of large, invasive lesions can lead to significant disfigurement and disability [53].

In infants, rhabdomyosarcoma (32.8%) is the most common malignant soft tissue tumor, followed in frequency by infantile fibrosarcoma (24.5%) and rhabdoid tumors (14.2%) [53]. Overall, malignant soft tissue tumors are rare in neonates. Rhabdoid tumors represent rare, aggressive malignancies that typically occur not only in the kidney and brain but can also be found in various soft tissue locations [54]. These tumors are relatively chemoresistant, demonstrate early tumor recurrence following surgical resection, and portend an overall poor prognosis [54].

9. Birth considerations

Certain neonatal tumors warrant special consideration regarding fetal delivery and perinatal management. Neoplasms that compromise the fetal airway represent an immediate threat to the neonatal airway, with the potential for hypoxia, ischemic brain injury, and death [55]. Cervical teratomas, cervical lymphatic malformations, and cervical hemangiomas are the most common neoplasms with the propensity to cause extrinsic airway compression in the neck. Mediastinal tumors that compress the great vessels or intrathoracic trachea also demand specialized pre- and postnatal care. Large tumors, particularly sacrococcygeal teratomas, merit consideration for Cesarean or early delivery as a method to avoid intrauterine or perinatal complications.

Prior to the development of the ex utero intrapartum treatment (EXIT) procedure, case reports described managing obstructing cervical masses with bronchoscopy and intubation prior to division of the umbilical cord [56]. The operation on placental support (OOPS) procedure involved Cesarean delivery of the head and thorax in order to perform endotracheal intubation [57]. Inhaled isoflurane anesthesia was administered in hopes of minimizing uterine contractions in an effort to preserve fetoplacental circulation and prevent placental abruption [57]. These early procedures were felt to provide inadequate tocolysis and/or reduce the uterine volume through fetal delivery, both of which result in uterine contraction and interruption of uteroplacental gas exchange [58].

Currently, the EXIT procedure offers a more comprehensive management approach to fetal and neonatal airway obstruction. The procedure also has application in the treatment of pulmonary and mediastinal masses leading to airway obstruction or other physiologic derangements. The EXIT procedure [59] entails intubating the mother and administering deep inhalational anesthesia with high-dose (2–3%) isoflurane. Anesthetic alone provides adequate uterine relaxation in many cases, but bolus doses of terbutaline or nitroglycerin can be given when necessary. Prior to performing hysterotomy, ultrasound is used to identify the location of the fetus and placenta. Following hysterotomy, the head and thorax of the fetus are delivered, allowing for multiple procedures to be performed, including bronchoscopy, orotracheal intubation, tracheostomy, mass excision, and ECMO cannulation. Fetoplacental circulation is preserved during the procedure and mitigates the possibility of hypoxia and brain ischemia. Once the airway is secured, the umbilical cord is divided, and Pitocin is administered, while the concentration of inhalational anesthetic is decreased to low levels or discontinued. The remainder of the procedure proceeds as would be expected from a routine Cesarean section.

Mediastinal tumors of appropriate size and location have the potential to cause fetal and neonatal demise through several mechanisms. One potential presentation is fetal airway and esophageal obstruction leading to polyhydramnios and preterm labor [60]. A second presentation is great vessel compression with resulting nonimmune fetal hydrops and fetal demise [60]. Several successful management strategies have been reported. One strategy involves aspiration of the cystic component of mediastinal teratomas for size reduction and alleviation of fetal hydrops until delivery and definitive management [61]. Serial amniocenteses to reduce uterine volume followed by neonatal resection have also been reported [60, 62–64].

http://dx.doi.org/10.5772/68070

The EXIT procedure also serves as a useful adjunct in transitioning these children from intrauterine life to definitive airway control, ECMO cannulation, or surgical resection.

10. Common specific lesions

10.1. Teratomas

Teratomas are the most common neonatal tumors, accounting for up to 30% of these lesions in some series [1, 20, 21]. Teratomas typically occur in the midline, spanning a variety of locations from the pineal gland to the coccyx [34]. The distribution of these tumors is explained by the fact that they arise from pluripotent germ cells that arrest in abnormal locations during embryologic migration [30]. Persistent division by these aberrant nests of cells results in tumors of varying size in diverse locations.

These neoplasms include all three germ cell layers, endoderm, mesoderm, and ectoderm. Most tumors are benign and can be classified as mature or immature based on their histologic appearance. Elements of the ectoderm, particularly neural tissue, are a dominant feature of immature fetal and neonatal teratomas [65, 66]. Mature and immature teratomas also contain mesenchymal components, including smooth muscle, cartilage, fat, and bone. Endodermal features such as respiratory and gastrointestinal epithelium are much less common [33, 65, 66]. Sacrococcygeal teratomas are the most common type of these tumors, followed in frequency by intracranial, cervical, palatal and nasopharyngeal, cardiac, gastric, and mediastinal teratomas [33]. Survival rates vary considerably by location, with intracranial teratomas (11%) having the lowest survival and gastric teratomas (100%) demonstrating the best prognosis [33].

Sacrococcygeal teratomas represent 40–60% of teratomas and demonstrate a 3 to 1 female to male distribution [33, 67]. The estimated incidence is 1 in every 35,000 live births [68]. In countries where prenatal ultrasound is ubiquitous, many lesions are diagnosed in utero. In the absence of prenatal diagnosis, the classic presentation is that of a newborn with an evident mass on physical examination. Diagnosis of purely pelvic teratomas is frequently delayed [69]. Children in this category may develop urinary retention, constipation, a palpable abdominal mass, or failure to thrive. MRI serves as a useful adjunct to ultrasound in determining the degree of intrapelvic extension. In 1973, Altman et al. [69] developed a location-based classification system for sacrococcygeal teratoma. Type I tumors are mainly external (sacrococcygeal) with minimal presacral component. Type II tumors exhibit an external component on presentation but have a substantial intrapelvic component. Type III tumor indicates a tumor with minimal external component with the majority of the mass located intrapelvic and extending into the abdomen. Type IV tumors are found entirely in the presacral space without any external component. Accurate classification is critical to parental counseling and appropriate operative planning.

Large sacrococcygeal teratomas represent a challenging diagnosis due to their potential to cause perinatal complications as well as unpredictable growth patterns [70]. Potential complications associated with these tumors are numerous, consisting of premature labor from polyhydramnios or increased intrauterine volume, tumor rupture, labor dystocia, hemorrhage, maternal mirror syndrome, and fetal hydrops secondary to high-output cardiac failure in highly vascular lesions [70]. Prenatally diagnosed sacrococcygeal teratomas should undergo frequent surveillance to monitor for rapidity of growth and development of the aforementioned complications [63]. For tumors that demonstrate a predominantly solid component with high vascularity, open fetal surgery may be necessary for tumor debulking to prevent high-output cardiac failure and fetal hydrops [71]. Similar to the management options for mediastinal teratomas, cyst aspiration and serial amniocenteses are beneficial interventions in appropriately selected patients [63, 64]. Cesarean delivery should be considered in larger lesions to prevent labor dystocia, tumor rupture, and hemorrhage.

En bloc resection of the tumor and coccyx is the primary treatment modality for sacrococcygeal teratoma. Failure to remove the coccyx and gross tumor spillage appear to have the highest association with recurrence [72]. The presence of microscopically positive margins necessitates routine surveillance in the absence of yolk sac tumor elements on final pathology, while histologic confirmation of yolk sac tumor components warrants adjuvant chemotherapy [72]. The age at diagnosis correlates with the presence of underlying malignancy and overall survival. Approximately 10% of neonatal sacrococcygeal teratomas contain a yolk sac tumor with the incidence of a concurrent malignancy increasing with age [33]. The outcome of fetuses diagnosed with sacrococcygeal teratoma is worse than those diagnosed in neonates. The estimated mortality for prenatally diagnosed lesions ranges from 33 to 50% and approaches 100% when fetal hydrops is present [33, 63, 73]. Conversely, the survival for a newborn diagnosed with this disease approaches 90% following complete surgical excision [33, 63, 73].

10.2. Neuroblastoma

Neuroblastoma represents the second most common neonatal tumor, accounting for 22.5–30% of these neoplasms, and the most common congenital malignancy [1, 20, 21]. Neuroblastomas are derived from primitive neural crest cells, or neuroblasts, and can be identified in any location where sympathetic tissue exists [74, 75]. Nearly 90% of fetal and neonatal cases of neuroblastoma occur in the adrenal gland compared to 35% in infants and older children [75, 76]. The next most common sites, in order to decrease frequency, are the retroperitoneum, posterior mediastinum, and neck [32]. The incidence of neuroblastoma is approximately 1 in 100,000 children, with a mean age of diagnosis of 18 months [77]. The incidence of neuroblastoma in neonates is not as well defined as tumors occur less commonly in this age group compared to older children.

Neuroblastoma is being diagnosed with increased frequency on prenatal ultrasound due to widespread use of fetal sonography and continued technological improvement [78]. In fact, there was once an interest in screening for neuroblastoma with prenatal ultrasound, but in general this practice has been abandoned as it only succeeded in identifying lesions that could otherwise be observed and did not identify the more aggressive lesions that most are interested in identifying early. The differential diagnosis of an adrenal lesion includes adrenal hemorrhage, adrenal abscess, adrenal cyst, and renal anomalies. Nearly all cases are diagnosed during the third trimester. Identification of a solid or cystic adrenal mass should

http://dx.doi.org/10.5772/68070

raise suspicion for the presence of an underlying neuroblastoma [78]. Postnatal MRI serves as useful to clarify the extent of disease and guide treatment options. Most mothers with a prenatal diagnosis of neuroblastoma are asymptomatic, although maternal hypertension and preeclampsia may occur due to elevated levels of catecholamines in maternal circulation [76]. In the absence of a prenatal diagnosis of neuroblastoma, presentation is variable and includes detection of a palpable abdominal mass, hepatomegaly, respiratory distress, and the presence of cutaneous nodules. Neuroblastomas are hormonally active tumors that secrete high levels of catecholamines and their by-products. The diagnosis can be further solidified by detection of these chemicals in a urine sample, although serum levels are not predictive of prognosis and do not dictate treatment.

Staging of neuroblastoma follows the International Neuroblastoma Staging System, which considers tumor location, nodal involvement, and the presence of metastases in assessing the burden of disease [79]. The majority of fetal and neonatal cases of neuroblastoma are stage I, stage II, and stage IV-S at the time of diagnosis [32, 76, 77]. Most tumors also demonstrate favorable histology including N-myc non-amplification, stroma-rich appearance, and aneuploid DNA content [32, 76, 77]. Surgical resection is the principal treatment for localized cases of neuroblastoma. In cases of unresectable disease, open or core needle biopsy provides valuable histologic information to help guide treatment decisions. Neonates with stage IV-S represent a particularly unique group of patients who have a localized tumor with metastases isolated to the liver, bone, and skin [79]. Despite the presence of metastatic disease, these children have a favorable prognosis, and many tumors undergo spontaneous regression without specific treatment. Treatment options for stage IV-S include observation, surgical resection, and chemotherapy. Chemotherapy is also employed in the neoadjuvant setting for tumors that are initially deemed to be unresectable. Overall, the prognosis for fetal and neonatal neuroblastoma is excellent, with survival ranging from 70 to 100% [32, 76, 77]. There have been favorable studies that have demonstrated success with observation with small lesions that likely represent neuroblastoma [80]. Moving forward, current staging is changing from a surgery-based staging toward image-defined risk categories with the majority of neonatal lesions falling into the low-risk categories. Therefore, we would recommend that these patients should be enrolled in current observation studies to document outcomes of this patient population.

10.3. Infantile hepatic hemangioma and mesenchymal hamartoma

Infantile hepatic hemangiomas are the most common primary liver tumors in newborns. Hemangiomas display a wide range of behavior, spanning from asymptomatic masses to those causing significant physiologic distress and potential demise [41]. Most lesions are diagnosed on prenatal imaging or found incidentally on physical examination. In some cases, the presence of cutaneous hemangiomas prompts evaluation for a concomitant hepatic mass [41]. Infantile hepatic hemangiomas are benign, vascular masses characterized by rapid postnatal growth followed by involution in childhood [42]. For this reason, asymptomatic and smaller lesions can be observed for involution through serial ultrasonography. Conversely, some lesions develop severe arteriovenous shunting, which can lead to high-output cardiac failure, fetal hydrops, and death. Other masses lead to Kasabach-Merritt syndrome, which can cause consumptive coagulopathy, thrombocytopenia, and hemolytic anemia [81]. Surgical excision is an effective management for localized lesions in children without severe physiologic derangement. Selective hepatic arterial embolization can be used to induce preoperative tumor shrinkage and in cases of refractory coagulopathy [82].

Mesenchymal hamartomas are the second most common hepatic tumor in newborns. These lesions are congenital malformations that contain elements of normal hepatic parenchyma including mesenchyme, portal venous branches, bile ducts, hepatocytes, and cysts of varying size [41]. Hamartomas are benign masses that display several chromosomal abnormalities [83]. Similar to hemangiomas, hamartomas are typically identified on prenatal imaging or found as an asymptomatic mass on physical examination. Approximately 75% are found in the right hepatic lobe with the rest involving the left lobe or both lobes [84]. Although these are histologically benign tumors, some lesions demonstrate rapid growth and result in significant physiologic disturbance. Tumors abutting the diaphragm can cause significant respiratory compromise. Compression of intra-abdominal vascular structures may lead to nonimmune fetal hydrops and fetal demise. Complete surgical excision is the optimal management for children with hepatic mesenchymal hamartomas. In tumors with large cystic components, fetal aspiration has been reported to mitigate detrimental fetal and obstetric sequelae [85].

10.4. Ovarian cysts

Ovarian cysts are the most common masses identified in neonatal girls and are nearly always benign. The etiology of ovarian cysts is not completely understood, but hormonal stimulation is felt to be responsible for this disease process [86]. In 1975, Valenti et al. [87] reported the first case of a prenatally diagnosed ovarian cyst. With improvement in ultrasonography, ovarian cysts are being identified with increasing frequency on prenatal imaging. Ultrasound provides vital information about size, location, wall characteristics, and vascularity [41]. However, many lesions are asymptomatic and would not be identified if not for routine fetal ultrasound [88].

Treatment of ovarian cysts hinges upon the risk of complications and the ability to differentiate between truly benign cysts and other ovarian neoplasms [89]. The most common complication encountered is ovarian torsion with subsequent loss of the affected ovary [86, 89]. Many cases of ovarian torsion occur prenatally, precluding the ability to intervene in an effort for ovarian preservation. Doppler evaluation is an unreliable measure of torsion in this patient population secondary to vessel size and the fact that normal flow does not exclude the diagnosis [86]. Fetal cyst aspiration is one management strategy used to mitigate the risk of in utero torsion, but there is no agreed upon size cutoff to determine when this measure should be employed.

Simple cysts less than 4–5 cm in size can be observed for spontaneous regression with serial ultrasonography [41, 86, 88, 89]. Cysts larger than 4–5 cm are candidates for cyst aspiration or surgical intervention given a higher potential for ovarian torsion [41, 86, 88, 89]. Complex ovarian cysts, cysts that fail to regress spontaneously, cysts that recur following aspiration, and those that are symptomatic should be removed surgically [89]. Preservation of ovarian parenchyma is the hallmark of surgery for ovarian cysts. Options for surgical management include cyst unroofing, partial or total cystectomy, and oophorectomy. In cases of ovarian torsion, the macroscopic appearance of the ovary does not necessarily correlate with the degree of parenchymal damage [88]. Pathologic evaluation of a portion of the cyst wall is recommended; however, the presence of an underlying malignancy is exceedingly rare.

10.5. Cervical lymphatic malformations

Lymphatic malformations are characterized by localized collections of malformed lymphatic channels that occur most commonly in the head and neck [90]. Lymphatic malformations typically occur in the posterior neck and are often associated with karyotypic abnormalities [91]. Other common locations are the trunk and extremities, the thoracic cavity, and the abdominal cavity. Traditionally, lymphatic malformations have been assigned to different categories based on histologic appearance: cavernous lymphangiomas, capillary lymphangiomas, and cystic hygroma [90]. However, the histologic classification does not seem to correlate with clinical behavior or response to therapy [90]. These masses follow a variable clinical course, with prenatally diagnosed lesions having a worse prognosis than those identified following birth [91].

Lymphatic malformations typically grow proportionally with the growth of the child, with rapid enlargement occurring as the result of trauma, hemorrhage, or infection [91]. Spontaneous infection occurs in approximately 7–30% of these masses [92]. The size and location of a given lymphatic malformation are predictive of potential adverse consequences to the developing child. Head and neck lesions can lead to fetal esophageal obstruction, resulting in polyhydramnios and preterm labor. A more serious complication is the potential for neonatal airway obstruction and rapid demise following birth. The EXIT procedure [56] offers a comprehensive management strategy to establish a definitive airway while maintaining fetoplacental circulation. However, if the lesion is soft and away from the midline, such fetuses may not require EXIT as obtaining an airway may not be difficult. Intrathoracic lymphatic malformations also have the potential to cause airway obstruction. Compression of the great vessels in the thorax and abdomen can cause high-output cardiac failure, hydrops fetalis, and fetal demise.

Many treatment modalities exist for the management of lymphatic malformations. In general, asymptomatic lesions can be observed for some time as many of these lesions will resolve without intervention. In those lesions that are large, growing, or symptomatic, therapeutic maneuvers include sclerotherapy and surgery. Prior to pursuing these therapies, the extent of the tumor and association with surrounding structures must be determined [91]. Nerves and major vessels should be preserved [90]. More complex and invasive lesions may require multiple, staged operations to achieve complete resection [90, 91]. Tumors that undergo complete macroscopic excision show the lowest recurrence rates but still return in 17% of cases [93]. Recurrences occur in up to 100% of cases following aspiration and in 40% of masses that are incompletely excised [93]. The estimated recurrence rate following injection of sclerosing agents, such as sodium tetradecanol, bleomycin, and OK-432, ranges from 50 to 100% [91, 93]. Aspiration does play a role in emergent cases to decrease the mass effect of the tumor and establish an airway [90]. In small, asymptomatic lesions, a period of surveillance to monitor for spontaneous regression may also be pursued [90].

10.6. Rhabdomyosarcoma

Soft tissue tumors account for 8–12% of neonatal tumors [1, 20, 21]. Rhabdomyosarcoma is the most common malignant soft tissue tumor in children, representing one third of these masses in infants and nearly half of soft tissue tumors found in older children [53]. Rhabdomyosarcoma is an aggressive, embryonal tumor of childhood marked by high-grade histology, local invasiveness, and a propensity to metastasize [53]. There are two main histologic subtypes: embryonal rhabdomyosarcoma accounts for nearly 70% of all cases and portends a better prognosis and alveolar rhabdomyosarcoma which is characterized by numerous chromosomal translocations and has a worse overall outcome [94]. As mesenchymal tumors that arise from skeletal muscle, rhabdomyosarcoma can occur in many locations throughout the body. The most common sites of occurrence are the head and neck followed by the genitourinary system and extremities [53]. Neonatal cases of rhabdomyosarcoma are rare. Male gender, Caucasian race, embryonal subtype, and undifferentiated histology are the predominant characteristics in neonates [95].

Rhabdomyosarcoma may be identified on prenatal imaging but more commonly presents as an identifiable mass following birth. The differential diagnosis is broad and includes many benign and malignant soft tissue tumors. Lymphatic involvement and metastatic disease are present in nearly 20% of cases at presentation [53]. The most common sites of metastasis are the lung, bone marrow, and bone. Neonatal cases of alveolar rhabdomyosarcoma may present with brain metastases and subcutaneous nodules [96]. Biopsy of the primary lesion is recommended for diagnostic purposes and to determine tumor biology to guide treatment. However, one should proceed with complete excision of smaller lesions (<5 cm) if this can be performed with clear margins and without injury to surrounding structures. Larger or difficult to excise lesions should have an incisional biopsy with a sufficient tissue sample to allow for all necessary studies (1 cm^3). Following diagnosis, tumors require staging with CT or MRI of the primary lesion, imaging of the chest, bone marrow aspiration, and bone marrow biopsy.

Treatment of neonatal rhabdomyosarcomas should be undertaken in a multidisciplinary fashion. Therapy is multimodal and includes systemic chemotherapy for metastatic disease and surgical resection and radiation for local disease. Complete surgical resection may not always be feasible, and age at diagnosis dictates the ability to give chemotherapy and radiation. Age is an independent prognostic factor with children less than 1 year of age having a worse overall prognosis than children between the ages of 1 and 10 [97, 98]. In the Intergroup Rhabdomyosarcoma Study, Lobe et al. [95] found that only 49% of 14 newborns diagnosed with rhabdomyosarcoma were alive at 3 years.

10.7. Congenital mesoblastic nephroma

Congenital mesoblastic nephroma is the most common renal tumor occurring in neonates and during the first 3 months of life [45]. In a retrospective review of 210 renal tumors in fetuses and infants less than 2 months of age, Isaacs [44] found that the four most common renal neoplasms were congenital mesoblastic nephroma (66%), Wilms' tumor (20%), rhabdoid tumor of the kidney (11%), and clear cell sarcoma of the kidney (3%). Congenital mesoblastic nephroma demonstrates a slight male predominance with a male to female ratio of 1.5 to 1 [45]. The most common presentations of mesoblastic nephroma are prenatal identification on fetal ultrasound, polyhydramnios, and palpation of an abdominal mass following birth. Sonographically, the presence of an anechoic circle or "ring sign" surrounding the mass may help differentiate congenital mesoblastic nephroma from other renal neoplasms [46]. These tumors typically demonstrate benign behavior; however, in addition to polyhydramnios, some masses may be complicated by hypertension; respiratory compromise; circulatory compromise from large, space-occupying lesions; and fetal hydrops [44].

Congenital mesoblastic nephroma (CMN) is a benign neoplasm that is characterized by leiomyomatous histology with bundles of spindle cells, rare mitoses, and lack of necrosis [99]. The tumor can be further subdivided into classic and cellular subtypes based on histological appearance. Patients with the cellular subtype of CMN tend to have larger tumor burdens and older age of presentation [99]. Additionally, many cellular mesoblastic nephromas are cystic in nature, which may lead to increased risk of rupture and higher rates of recurrence [99]. Radical nephrectomy is the mainstay of treatment for a neonate diagnosed with CMN. Patients with the classic subtype of CMN are typically cured with surgical excision alone, while aggressive tumors, which are often of the cellular subtype, may require adjuvant chemotherapy. Recurrence occurs in 5% of patients, while metastases are present in 2% of cases [44]. The overall survival for a patient diagnosed with congenital mesoblastic nephroma is 95–98% [99, 100].

11. Chemotherapy and irradiation

One of the greatest challenges in pediatric oncology is determining the appropriate dosing regimen for chemotherapeutic agents in young children [101]. Multiple factors influence the pharmacology of chemotherapeutic drugs in the newborn, including changes in blood flow, hepatic and renal development, and alterations in the amount of body composition attributed to fat and water [101]. Body surface area dosing is the most commonly employed dosing method in the pediatric setting, but there are inconsistencies in the cutoffs and magnitude for dose reductions [101]. Administration of chemotherapy in newborns should always take place under the guidance of a pediatric oncologist.

Radiation therapy is also very challenging in the pediatric patient population. Although radiation therapy has been successful in the treatment of many pediatric cancers, concerns remain about long-term side effects [102]. Growth and development failure is a primary concern for children who receive radiation therapy [102]. Other late sequelae include neurocognitive defects, infertility, cardiac and pulmonary abnormalities, gastrointestinal dysfunction, and secondary cancer development [102]. Over the last 35 years, the use of radiation therapy has declined in the treatment of many pediatric cancers, including Wilms' tumor, neuroblastoma, ALL, and non-Hodgkin's lymphoma [102]. The decision to use radiation therapy in the treatment of neonatal tumors should always include a discussion of the risks and benefits of therapy with a radiation oncologist. Of note for this patient population is the need to perform radiation under sedation as the drugs used in this treatment modality are under investigation as to potential long-term side effects.

12. Conclusion

Neonatal tumors encompass an extremely diverse, heterogeneous group of neoplasms. Neonatal tumors demonstrate a broad spectrum of behaviors and outcomes with some lesions spontaneously regressing without treatment, while others are resistant to aggressive, multimodal therapy. The majority of lesions are benign, but histologic classification is not always predictive of clinical behavior or overall outcome. Treatment of neonatal tumors requires a clear understanding of the natural history of disease and the limitations of each treatment modality. The optimal management strategy incorporates the expertise of pediatricians, pediatric surgeons, pediatric medical oncologists, and pediatric radiation oncologists.

Author details

Kenneth W. Gow* and Matthew Dellinger

*Address all correspondence to: kenneth.gow@seattlechildrens.org

Seattle Children's Hospital and the University of Washington, USA

References

[1] Moore SW, Satge D, Sasco AJ, et al. The epidemiology of neonatal tumours. Report of an international working group. Pediatric Surgery International. 2003;**19**:509–519

[2] Weitzman S, Grant R. Neonatal oncology: Diagnostic and therapeutic dilemmas. Seminars in Perinatology. 1997;**21**(1):102–111

[3] Batcup G. Cancer in the very young child—pitfalls and problems for the pathologist. British Journal of Cancer. Supplement. 1992;**18**:S5-S7

[4] Halperin E. Neonatal neoplasms. International Journal of Radiation Oncology Biology Physics. 2000;**47**(1):171–178

[5] Orbach D, Sarnacki S, Brisse HJ, et al. Neonatal cancer. Lancet Oncology. 2013;**14**:e609-e620

[6] Merks JHM, Caron HN, Hennekam RCM. High incidence of malformation syndromes in a series of 1073 children with cancer. American Journal of Medical Genetics. 2005;**134**:132–143

[7] Santos XM, Papanna R, Johnson A, et al. The use of combined ultrasound and magnetic resonance imaging in the detection of fetal anomalies. Prenatal Diagnosis. 2010;**30**:402–407

[8] Nemec SF, Horcher E, Kasprian G, et al. Tumor disease and associated congenital abnormalities on prenatal MRI. European Journal of Radiology. 2012;**81**:e115-e122

[9] Lee TC, Olutoye OO. Evaluation of the prenatally diagnosed mass. Seminars in Fetal & Neonatal Medicine. 2012;**17**:185–191

[10] Pugash D, Brugger PC, Bettelheim D, et al. Prenatal ultrasound and fetal MRI: The comparative value of each modality in prenatal diagnosis. European Journal of Radiology. 2008;**68**:214–226

[11] Chung R, Kasprian G, Brugger PC, et al. The current state and future of fetal imaging. Clinics in Perinatology. 2009;**36**:685–699

[12] Bricker L, Garcia J, Henderson J, et al. Ultrasound screening in pregnancy: A systematic review of the clinical effectiveness, cost-effectiveness, and women's views. Health Technology Assessment. 2000;**4**(16):1–193

[13] Chen MM, Coakley FV, Kaimal A, et al. Guideline for computed tomography and magnetic resonance imaging use during pregnancy and lactation. Obstetrics & Gynecology. 2008;**112**:333–340

[14] Breysem L, Bosmans H, Dymarkowski S, et al. The value of fast MR imaging as an adjunct to ultrasound in prenatal diagnosis. European Radiology. 2003;**13**:1538–1548

[15] Wagenvoort AM, Bekker MN, Go ATJI, et al. Ultrafast scan magnetic resonance in prenatal diagnosis. Fetal Diagnosis and Therapy. 2000;**15**:364–372

[16] American College of Obstetricians and Gynecologists' Committee on Obstetric Practice. Guidelines for diagnostic imaging during pregnancy and lactation. Obstetrics & Gynecology. 2016;**127**(2):e75-e80

[17] Kanal E, Barkovich AJ, Bell C, et al. ACR guidance document on MR safe practices: 2013. Expert Panel on MR Safety. Journal of Magnetic Resonance Imaging. 2013;**37**:501–530

[18] Alamo L, Beck-Popovic M, Gudinchet F, et al. Congenital tumors: Imaging when life just begins. Insights into Imaging. 2011;**2**:297–308

[19] Borsellino A, Zaccara A, Nahom A, et al. False-positive rate in prenatal diagnosis of surgical anomalies. Journal of Pediatric Surgery. 2006;**41**:826–829

[20] Isaacs H Jr. Congenital and neonatal malignant tumors. A 28-year experience at Children's Hospital of Los Angeles. The American Journal of Pediatric Hematology/Oncology. 1987;**9**(2):121–129

[21] Parkes SE, Muir KR, Southern L, et al. Neonatal tumours: A thirty-year population-based study. Medical and Pediatric Oncology. 1994;**22**:309–317

[22] Bauchet L, Rigau V, Mathieu-Daudé H, et al. Clinical epidemiology for childhood primary central nervous system tumors. Journal of Neuro-Oncology. 2009;**92**:87–98

[23] Ostrom QT, Gittleman H, Fulop J, et al. CBTRUS statistical report: Primary brain and central nervous system tumors diagnosed in the United States in 2008–2012. Neuro-Oncology. 2015;**17**:iv1-iv62

[24] Isaacs H Jr. Perinatal brain tumors: A review of 250 cases. Pediatric Neurology. 2002; **27**:333–342

[25] Magdum SA. Neonatal brain tumours—a review. Early Human Development. 2010;**86**: 627–631

[26] Goins MR, Beasley MS. Pediatric neck masses. Oral & Maxillofacial Surgery Clinics of North America. 2012;**24**:457–468

[27] Torsiglieri AJ Jr, Tom LWC, Ross AJ III, et al. Pediatric neck masses: Guidelines for evaluation. International Journal of Pediatric Otorhinolaryngology. 1988;**16**:199

[28] Krol A, MacArthur CJ. Congenital hemangiomas: Rapidly involuting and noninvoluting congenital hemangiomas. Archives of Facial Plastic Surgery. 2005:**7**:307–311

[29] Kanada KN, Merin MR, Munden A, et al. A prospective study of cutaneous findings in newborns in the United States: Correlation with race, ethnicity, and gestational status using updated classification and nomenclature. Journal of Pediatrics. 2012;**161**:240–245

[30] Tranvinh E, Yeom KW, Iv M. Imaging neck masses in the neonate and young infant. Seminars in Ultrasound, CT, and MRI. 2015;**36**:120–137

[31] Dickson PV, Davidoff AM. Malignant neoplasms of the head and neck. Seminars in Pediatric Surgery. 2006;**15**(2):92–98

[32] Isaacs H Jr. Fetal and neonatal neuroblastoma: Retrospective review of 271 cases. Fetal and Pediatric Pathology. 2007;**26**:177–184

[33] Isaacs H Jr. Perinatal (fetal and neonatal) germ cell tumors. Journal of Pediatric Surgery. 2004;**39**(7):1003–1013

[34] Woodward PJ, Sohaey R, Kennedy A, Koeller KK. From the archives of the AFIP: A comprehensive review of fetal tumors with pathologic correlation. Radiographics. 2005;**25**(1):215–242

[35] Wienk MA, Van Geijn HP, Copray FJ, Brons JT. Prenatal diagnosis of fetal tumors by ultrasonography. Obstetrical & Gynecological Survey. 1990;**45**:639–653

[36] Isaacs H Jr. Fetal and neonatal cardiac tumors. Pediatric Cardiology. 2004;**25**:252–273

[37] Chan HS, Sonley MJ, Moes CA, Daneman A, Smith CR, Martin DJ. Primary and secondary tumors of childhood involving the heart, pericardium, and great vessels. A report of 75 cases and review of the literature. Cancer. 1985;**56**:825–836

[38] Van der Hauwaert LG. Cardiac tumours in infancy and childhood. British Heart Journal. 1971;**33**:125–132

[39] Jaggers J, Balsara K. Mediastinal masses in children. Seminars in Thoracic and Cardiovascular Surgery. 2004;**16**:201–208

[40] Priest JR, Williams MG, Hill DA, et al. Pulmonary cysts in early childhood and the risk of malignancy. Pediatric Pulmonology. 2009;**44**:14–30

[41] Chandler JC, Gauderer MWL. The neonate with an abdominal mass. Pediatric Clinics of North America. 2004;**51**:979–997

[42] Isaacs H Jr. Fetal and neonatal hepatic tumors. Journal of Pediatric Surgery. 2007; **42**:1797–1803

[43] Trobaugh-Lotrario AD, Chaiyachati BH, Meyers RL, et al. Outcomes for patients with congenital hepatoblastoma. Pediatric Blood & Cancer. 2013;**60**:1817–1825

[44] Isaacs H Jr. Fetal and neonatal renal tumors. Journal of Pediatric Surgery. 2008;**43**: 1587–1595

[45] Powis M. Neonatal renal tumors. Early Human Development. 2010;**86**:607–612

[46] Kelner M, Droullé P, Didier F, et al. The vascular "ring" sign in mesoblastic nephroma: Report of two cases. Pediatric Radiology. 2003;**33**:123–128

[47] Manivel JC. Testicular germ cell tumors (TGCTs) in neonates and infants. Seminars in Diagnostic Pathology. 2016;**33**(6):410–148

[48] Ross JH. Prepubertal testicular tumors. Urology. 2008;**74**:94–99

[49] Ross J, Rybicki L, Kay R. Clinical behavior and a contemporary management algorithm for prepubertal testis tumors: A summary of the Prepubertal Testis Tumor Registry. Journal of Urology. 2002;**168**:1675–1679

[50] Quint EH, Smith YR. Ovarian surgery in premenarchal girls. Journal of Pediatric & Adolescent Gynecology. 1999;**12**:27–30

[51] Navarro OM, Laffan EE, Ngan BY. Pediatric soft-tissue tumors and pseudotumors: MRI imaging features with pathologic correlation. Radiographics. 2009;**29**:887–906

[52] Bruyeer E, Lemmerling M, Poorten VV, et al. Paediatric lipoblastoma in the head and neck: Three cases and review of literature. Cancer Imaging. 2012;**12**:484–487

[53] Ferrari A, Orbach D, Sultan I, et al. Neonatal soft tissue sarcomas. Seminars in Fetal & Neonatal Medicine. 2012;**17**:231–238

[54] Bourdeaut F, Fréneaux P, Thuille B, et al. Extra-renal non-cerebral rhabdoid tumours. Pediatric Blood & Cancer. 2008;**51**:363–368

[55] Marwan A, Crombleholme TM. The EXIT procedure: Principles, pitfalls, and progress. Seminars in Pediatric Surgery. 2006;**15**:107–115

[56] Langer JC, Tabb T, Thompson P, et al. Management of prenatally diagnosed tracheal obstruction: Access to the airway in utero prior to delivery. Fetal Diagnosis and Therapy. 1992;**7**:12–16

[57] Skarsgard ED, Chitkara U, Krane EJ, et al. The OOPS procedure (operation on placental support): In utero airway management of the fetus with prenatally diagnosed tracheal obstruction. Journal of Pediatric Surgery. 1996;**31**:826–828

[58] McNamara H, Johnson N. The effect of uterine contractions on fetal oxygen saturation. British Journal of Obstetrics and Gynaecology. 1995;**102**:644–647

[59] Mychaliska GB, Bealer JF, Graf JL, et al. Operating on placental support: The ex utero intrapartum treatment procedure. Journal of Pediatric Surgery. 1997;**32**:227–231

[60] Merchant AM, Hedrick HL, Johnson MP, et al. Management of fetal mediastinal teratoma. Journal of Pediatric Surgery. 2005;**40**:228–231

[61] Takayasu H, Kitano Y, Kuroda T, et al. Successful management of a large fetal mediastinal teratoma complicated by hydrops fetalis. Journal of Pediatric Surgery. 2010;**45**: e21-e24

[62] Dumbell HR, Coleman AC, Pudifin JM, et al. Prenatal ultrasonographic diagnosis and successful management of mediastinal teratoma. A case report. South African Medical Journal. 1990;**20**:481–483

[63] Hedrick HL, Flake AW, Crombleholme TM, et al. Sacrococcygeal teratoma; Prenatal assessment, fetal intervention, and outcome. Journal of Pediatric Surgery. 2004;**39**:430–438

[64] Makin EC, Hyett J, Ade-Ajayi N, et al. Outcome of antenatally diagnosed sacrococcygeal teratomas: Single-center experience (1993–2004). Journal of Pediatric Surgery. 2006;**41**:388–393

[65] Isaacs H Jr. Perinatal (congenital and neonatal) neoplasms: A report of 110 cases. Pediatric Pathology. 1985;**3**:165–216

[66] Werb P, Scurry J, Ostor A, et al. Survey of congenital tumors in perinatal necropsies. Pathology. 1992;**24**:247–253

[67] Billmire DF, Grosfeld JL. Teratomas of childhood: Analysis of 142 cases. Journal of Pediatric Surgery. 1986;**21**:548–551

[68] Pantoja E, Liobet R, Gonsales-Flores B. Retroperitoneal teratoma: Historic review. Journal of Urology. 1976;**115**:520–523

[69] Altmann RP, Randolph JG, Lilly JR. Sacrococcygeal teratoma: American Academy of Pediatrics Surgical Section Survey 1973. Journal of Pediatric Surgery. 1974;**9**:389–398

[70] Roybal JL, Moldenhauer JS, Khalek N, et al. Early delivery as an alternative management strategy for selected high-risk fetal sacrococcygeal teratomas. Journal of Pediatric Surgery. 2011;**46**: 1325–1332

[71] Adzick NS. Open fetal surgery for life-threatening fetal anomalies. Seminars in Fetal & Neonatal Medicine. 2010;**15**(1):1–8

[72] De Backer A, Madern GC, Hakvoort-Cammel FGAJ, et al. Study of the factors associated with recurrence in children with sacrococcygeal teratoma. Journal of Pediatric Surgery. 2006;**41**:173–181

[73] Holterman AX, Filiatrault D, Lallier M, et al. The natural history of sacrococcygeal teratomas diagnosed through routine obstetric sonogram: A single institution experience. Journal of Pediatric Surgery. 1998;**33**:899–903

[74] Fisher JPH, Tweddle DA. Neonatal neuroblastoma. Seminars in Fetal & Neonatal Medicine. 2012;**17**:207–215

[75] Lonergan GJ, Schwab CM, Suarez ES, et al. Neuroblastoma, ganglioneuroblastoma, and ganglioneuroma: Radiologic-pathologic correlation. Radiographics. 2002;**22**:911–934

[76] Acharya S, Jayabose S, Kogan SJ, et al. Prenatally diagnosed neuroblastoma. Cancer. 1997;**80**:304–310

[77] Kostyrka B, Li J, Soundappan SV, et al. Features and outcomes of neonatal neuroblastoma. Pediatric Surgery International. 2011;**27**:937–941

[78] Ho PTC, Estroff JA, Kozakewich M, et al. Prenatal detection of neuroblastoma. A ten year experience from the Dana Farber Cancer Institute and Children's Hospital. Pediatrics. 1993;**92**(3):358–364

[79] Brodeur GM, Pritchard J, Berthold F, et al. Revisions of the international criteria for neuroblastoma diagnosis, staging, and response to treatment. Journal of Clinical Oncology. 1993;**11**:1466–1467

[80] Nuchtern JG, London, WB, Barnewolt CE, et al. A prospective study of expectant observation as primary therapy for neuroblastoma in young infants: A Children's Oncology Group study. Annals of Surgery. 2012;**256**(4):573–580

[81] Haisley-Royster C, Enjolras O, Frieden IJ, et al. Kasabach-Merritt phenomenon: A retrospective study of treatment with vincristine. Journal of Pediatric Hematology/Oncology. 2002;**24**(6):459–462

[82] Kullendorff CM, Cwikiel W, Sandstrom S. Embolization of hepatic hemangiomas in infants. European Journal of Pediatric Surgery. 2002;**12**(5):348–352

[83] Murthi GV, Paterson L, Azmy A. Chromosomal translocation in mesenchymal hamartoma of liver: What is its significance? Journal of Pediatric Surgery. 2003;**38**(10):1543–1545

[84] Stringer MD, Alizai NK. Mesenchymal hamartoma of the liver: A systematic review. Journal of Pediatric Surgery. 2005;**40**:1681–1690

[85] Tsao K, Hirose S, Sydorak R, et al. Fetal therapy for giant hepatic cysts. Journal of Pediatric Surgery. 2002;**37**(10):e31

[86] Bagolan P, Giorlandino C, Nahom A, et al. The management of fetal ovarian cysts. Journal of Pediatric Surgery. 2002;**37**(1):25–30

[87] Valenti C, Kassner EG, Yermakov V, et al. Antenatal diagnosis of a fetal ovarian cyst. American Journal of Obstetrics and Gynecology. 1975;**123**:216–219

[88] Galinier P, Carfagna L, Juricic M, et al. Fetal ovarian cysts management and ovarian prognosis: A report of 82 cases. Journal of Pediatric Surgery. 2008;**43**:2004–2009

[89] Brandt ML, Luks FI, Filiatrault D, et al. Surgical indications in antenatally diagnosed ovarian cysts. Journal of Pediatric Surgery. 1991;**26**(3):276–282

[90] Bloom DC, Perkins JA, Manning SC. Management of lymphatic malformations. Current Opinion in Otolaryngology & Head and Neck Surgery. 2004;**12**:500–504

[91] Gallagher PG, Mahoney MJ, Gosche JR. Cystic hygroma in the fetus and newborn. Seminars in Perinatology. 1999;**23**(4):341–356

[92] Wiswell TE, Miller JA. Infections of congenital cervical neck masses associated with bacteremia. Journal of Pediatric Surgery. 1986;**21**:173–174

[93] Alqahtani A, Nguyen LT, Flageole H, et al. 25 years' experience with lymphangiomas in children. Journal of Pediatric Surgery. 1999;**34**(7):1164–1168

[94] De Giovanni C, Landuzzi L, Nicoletti G, et al. Molecular and cellular biology of rhabdomyosarcoma. Future Oncology. 2009;**5**:1449–1475

[95] Lobe TE, Wiener ES, Hays DM, et al. Neonatal rhabdomyosarcoma: The IRS experience. Journal of Pediatric Surgery. 1994;**29**:1167–1170

[96] Rodriguez-Galindo C, Hill DA, Onyekwere O, et al. Neonatal alveolar rhabdomyosarcoma with skin and brain metastases. Cancer. 2001;**92**:1613–1620

[97] Sultan I, Casanova M, Al-Jumaily U, et al. Soft tissue sarcomas in the first year of life. European Journal of Cancer. 2010;**46**:2449–2456

[98] Joshi D, Anderson JR, Paidas C, et al. Age is an independent prognostic factor in rhabdomyosarcoma: A report from the Soft Tissue Sarcoma Committee of the Children's Oncology Group. Pediatric Blood & Cancer. 2004;**42**(1):64–73

[99] Furtwaengler R, Reinhard H, Leuschner I, et al. Mesoblastic nephroma—a report from the Gesellschaft fur Pädiatrische Onkologie und Hämatologie (GPOH). Cancer. 2006;**106**:2275–2283

[100] Howell CG, Othersen HB, Kiviat NE, et al. Therapy and outcome in 51 children with mesoblastic nephroma: A report of the National Wilms' Tumor Study. Journal of Pediatric Surgery. 1982;**17**:826–831

[101] Veal GJ, Boddy AV. Chemotherapy in newborns and preterm babies. Seminars in Fetal and Neonatal Medicine. 2012;**17**(4):243–248

[102] Jairam V, Roberts KB, Yu JB. Historical trends in the use of radiation therapy for pediatric cancers: 1973–2008. International Journal of Radiation Oncology Biology Physics. 2013;**85**(3):e151-e155

Section 4

Pre and Postoperative Care of Pediatric Congenital Heart Disease

Pre and Postoperative Management of Pediatric Patients with Congenital Heart Diseases

Eva Miranda Marwali, Beatrice Heineking and
Nikolaus A. Haas

Additional information is available at the end of the chapter

http://dx.doi.org/10.5772/66990

Abstract

Stabilization during preoperative cardiac surgery especially in neonates has an important role to predict outcome for pediatric congenital heart surgery. We tried to elaborate general guidelines on how to diagnose and some anticipations for emergency treatments tailored by the type of congenital heart disease in neonates. Stabilization consists of medical treatment including emergent prostaglandin institution in some types of duct dependent lesion. The role of interventional catheterization such as patent ductus arteriosus (PDA) stent, balloon pulmonary valvotomy, etc. as modalities for stabilization before surgery was also elaborated. Some general and specific guidelines based on the type of surgeries for postoperative management were also discussed.

Keywords: pediatric, congenital heart disease, preoperative stabilization, postoperative management

1. Initial treatment of critically ill neonates with cardiac defects

In the following paragraphs of this chapter, the general features of various congenital heart defects, their clinical symptoms and treatment principles for the management of congenital heart defects that become symptomatic in neonates will be discussed. In this context, the special measures for the initial treatment of the most common defects are presented [1–8, 11].

1.1. Epidemiology

Based on many epidemiological studies, the actual incidence of congenital heart defects is 8–11 per 1000 live births independent of ethical background, social welfare or medical standards.

As a rule thumb nearly half of these children require any form of surgical or interventional intervention within the first year of life. With adequate management, more than 90% of these children can reach adulthood and lead a relatively normal life.

1.2. Symptoms

It is typical for the different congenital heart defects to present and become manifest at different times in early life. Of most importance are the very early phase when the patent ductus arteriosus closes for all ductal-dependent cardiac defects; the next important timeframe of clinical manifestation is the reduction in pulmonary vascular resistance (PVR) for defects with left-to-right shunt.

Note

Typical leading symptoms for the presentation of congenital heart defects in neonates are as follows:

- Heart failure or cardiogenic shock (usually in the first or second week of life if there is left heart obstruction; for shunt defects typically not until after the drop in pulmonary resistance at the age of 2–8 weeks)
- Cyanosis

Additional important clinical symptoms that may lead to the diagnosis of a congenital heart defect in neonates are the presence of a murmur on auscultation or any form of arrhythmia (rarely as the primary symptom of a congenital heart defect).

1.2.1. Heart failure

The characteristic clinical signs of heart failure in neonates are as follows:

- Tachypnea, dyspnea, thoracic retractions
- Rarely but possible pulmonary edema mainly due to overflow
- Tachycardia
- Hepatomegaly
- Failure to thrive, difficulty in feeding, increased sweating, abnormal sleepiness
- Pallor, prolonged capillary refill time

It is evident that the clinical symptoms of neonatal heart failure are unspecific and may be similar to the clinical symptoms of sepsis. Therefore, many neonates with heart failure are treated for suspected sepsis.

In particular, cardiac defects with left-sided obstruction (coarctation of the aorta, critical aortic stenosis, hypoplastic left heart syndrome), or typically become manifest as early as the first 1–2 weeks of life with the clinical symptoms of cardiogenic shock caused by early duct closure.

1.2.2. Cyanosis

- Cyanosis is a clinical sign that becomes evident when about 5% of the hemoglobin is deoxygenated. In neonates with polycythemia (Hb >20 g/dl), this may be present even without hypoxemia, in patients with anemia this may be overseen. To avoid this, pulse oximetry at all four limbs is the standard of care.
- *Neonatal screening*: Cyanosis in a newborn should be picked up by a neonatal screening program that measures saturation by pulse oximetry at all four extremities at the first day of life. It should be standard of care that all newborns should have this screening test. If the saturation is >95% and the control 12 h later is again >95%, a cyanotic heart defect can be ruled out. If the saturation is ≤95%, additional examinations (today—ECHO as the preferred method of choice) are needed.
- *Hyperoxia test*: The hyperoxia test is a more historical test and no longer useful in the times of ECHO. It was used to try and distinguish between cardiac and pulmonary cyanosis. In patients with pulmonary cyanosis, the oxygen saturation increases markedly after oxygen is given, while oxygen saturation is usually not significantly improved in those with cyanotic heart defects. This test lacks specificity and sensitivity to rule out or confirm cardiac defects. Both pre- and postductal oxygen saturation should be measured.
- Cardiac cyanosis can be the result of either reduced lung perfusion due to a right-to-left shunt, complete venous mixing in patients with total anomalous pulmonary venous return or intracardiac mixing of systemic and pulmonary venous blood. Methemoglobinemia is another rare cause for cyanosis. In addition, cyanosis can be caused by abnormality in the central nervous system (e.g., after cerebral hemorrhage or in cases with central apnea in premature neonates, etc.)

Note

All newborns should have a neonatal screening for congenital heart defects immediately after birth and 12 h later. Today ECHO is the main diagnostic tool for secondary investigation and to rule out or confirm congenital heart defects.

If the diagnosis can not be immediately confirmed by echocardiography, an attempt of treating the neonate with intravenous prostaglandin E1 is justified.

The hyperoxia test is no longer standard of care. If there is no adequate increase in oxygen saturation in a cyanosed neonate, a congenital heart defect with ductal dependent lung perfusion must be assumed.

1.2.3. Heart murmur

As innocent murmurs are unlikely in this age group, a heart murmur in a neonate is always suggestive of a congenital heart defect. Usually, stenosis of the semilunar valves or AV valve insufficiency present immediately after birth due to a loud systolic murmur, the typical VSD murmur in a large VSD, for example, can often be not auscultated until after the pulmonary resistance has dropped and the pressure gradient between the left and right ventricles increases. In addition, in many critical heart defects, there might be no indicative heart murmur at all (e.g., d-TGA simplex, coarctation of the aorta).

1.2.4. Arrhythmias

Arrhythmias often present in neonates without structural heart defects (i.e., atrial flutter, congenital AV block) and therefore are rarely the first symptom of a congenital heart defect. An AV block may occur in association with an l-TGA or heterotaxy syndromes. Supraventricular tachycardia due to accessory conduction pathways occurs more frequently with an Ebstein anomaly. The most common arrhythmia in a newborn is atrial flutter that requires immediate electrical cardioversion after diagnosis with adenosine but usually presents without additional defects.

1.3. Hemodynamic situation

The congenital heart defects that become symptomatic in neonates can be divided into five groups (**Table 1**).

Group	Examples
Cardiac defects with ductal-dependent systemic circulation (left heart obstructions)	Critical aortic stenosis, hypoplastic left heart syndrome, interrupted aortic arch, critical coarctation of the aorta
Cardiac defect with ductal-dependent pulmonary circulation (right heart obstructions)	Critical pulmonary stenosis, pulmonary atresia with intact ventricular septum, pulmonary atresia with VSD, pronounced form of Tetralogy of Fallot, severe Ebstein's anomaly, tricuspid atresia with pulmonary atresia or high-grade pulmonary stenosis
Cardiac defects with parallel circulation	d-TGA—transposition of the great arteries
Cardiac defects with complete intracardiac mixing of blood	Total anomalous pulmonary venous connection, univentricular heart
Cardiac defects with a large left-to-right shunt symptomatic usually after 4–6 weeks	Large VSD, complete AVSD, large PDA, aortopulmonary window, Truncus arteriosus communis, univentricular hearts with unobstructed pulmonary blood flow

Table 1. Classification of congenital heart defects which become symptomatic in the neonatal period.

In a ductal-dependent defect survival depends on the persistence of a patent ductus arteriosus. In general, ductal-dependent systemic circulation must be distinguished from ductal-dependent pulmonary circulation. In patients with ductal-dependent systemic circulation, there is a high-grade obstruction of the structures of the left heart (mitral valve, aortic valve, arch and coarctation). To ensure sufficient systemic perfusion, the systemic circulation must be supplied with blood from the pulmonary circulation across the patent ductus arteriosus like in utero. In ductal-dependent pulmonary circulation, there is a high-grade right heart obstruction leading to cyanosis. Perfusion of the pulmonary circulation depends mainly on the blood supply from the aorta across the patent ductus arteriosus.

In parallel circulations (d-TGA), survival depends on additional shunts (especially a sufficiently large atrial shunt) between the two circulations to enable mixing of the cyanosed and the arterialized blood.

http://dx.doi.org/10.5772/66990

In cardiac defects with complete intracardiac mixing of blood, the resulting cyanosis is often only relatively mild; when excessive pulmonary blood flow due to the lack of pulmonary stenosis is often present simultaneously, this leads to pulmonary recirculation of the saturated blood. Heart failure usually develops as a result of the excessive pulmonary blood flow after 4–6 weeks.

Based on this principle, congenital heart defects with a large left-to-right shunt do not become clinically symptomatic until the age of about 4–6 weeks; at that time, the PVR has dropped and the shunt between the systemic and pulmonary circulation increases dramatically. If left-sided heart obstruction is, however, also present (e.g., VSD with CoA), the symptoms may develop as early as the first week of life.

1.4. Diagnostic measures

1.4.1. Oxygen saturation

As a standard of care, oxygen saturation should always be measured in children both preductally (right hand) and postductally (lower limb). If there is a defect with ductal-dependent systemic circulation, the (postductal) oxygen saturation measured in the feet may be lower than the (preductal) saturation in the right hand.

The brachiocephalic trunk branches off from the aortic arch well before the ductus arteriosus; therefore, it is safe to assume that the saturation measured in the right hand is equivalent to preductal saturation (except in the rare cases of a lusoric artery).

1.4.2. Blood gas analysis (BGA)

As metabolic acidosis is the typical finding in severe heart failure and cardiogenic shock, routine (arterial) BGA is recommended on multiple occasions. In addition, all BGA should measure lactate as surrogate of cardiac output and thereby tissue perfusion.

1.4.3. Echocardiography (ECHO)

As mentioned before, today echocardiography is the diagnostic method of choice in all patients with a presumed cardiac defect or impaired circulatory situation. ECHO allows an accurate diagnosis of all significant cardiac defects that become symptomatic in the neonatal period. As modern standard of care, every neonatal unit must have ECHO and support of a pediatric cardiologist available on a 24/7 basis.

1.4.4. Hyperoxia test

In the time of ECHO, this test has only anecdotic relevance and lacks sensitivity and specificity. This test has been used to distinguish between cardiac or pulmonary central cyanosis. After breathing 100% oxygen for a few minutes, the cyanosis disappears or should be clearly reduced in pulmonary cyanosis and there is a relevant increase in arterial partial oxygen pressure. In cardiac cyanosis, the partial oxygen pressure should remain largely unchanged as the cardiac right-to-left shunt or inadequate pulmonary perfusion cannot be compensated by the administration of oxygen.

Note

Today in any case, echocardiography examination is preferable to a hyperoxia test and must be available in every neonatal unit on a 24/7 basis.

1.4.5. Pulse and blood pressure in all limbs

All neonates with suspected cardiac defect should have a pulse and blood pressure measurement at all 4 limbs. If a difference in blood pressure between the right arm (preductal) and the lower limbs (postductal) is then manifest or the peripheral pulses in the lower limbs cannot be palpated, this is a hint and leading findings of coarctation of the aorta or an interrupted aortic arch. This examination is helpful to assess systemic circulation.

Note

In a large patent ductus arteriosus, there may be no difference in blood pressure between the upper and lower halves of the body even with relevant coarctation of the aorta or interrupted aortic arch. The saturations, however, vary substantially.

1.5. Treatment

According to the different anatomic variations and physiologic situation, there is a substantial difference in the management of these children. The treatment principles for the various groups of congenital heart defects are presented below and based on the pathophysiology, the specific treatments of the individual heart defects in the neonatal period are described in this context.

1.5.1. Cardiac defects with ductal-dependent systemic circulation

In ductal-dependent systemic circulation, we should reestablish the prenatal circulation. Therefore, attempts must be made to provide as much blood as possible from the pulmonary circulation to supply the systemic circulation via the patent ductus arteriosus. As a result of this strategy, a saturation of 75–85% is adequate and saturations >85% that indicate excessive pulmonary blood flow should be avoided. The treatment principles of ductal-dependent systemic circulation are as follows:

- Provide patency of the ductus arteriosus with a continuous prostaglandin E1 infusion (initial dosage 20–50 ng/kg/min, to be reduced after ECHO assessment; caveat: Apnoea).
- Lower systemic vascular resistance:
    - By reducing afterload: i.e., with sodium nitroprusside infusion
    - If catecholamines are needed: Use preferably milrinone and/or dobutamine (vasodilatation effects); avoid vasoconstrictive effects of other catecholamines (dopamine, noradrenaline)

- Increase pulmonary resistance, increase pulmonary artery pressure:
  - Avoid intubation, extubate early
  - Avoid additional oxygen
  - Aim for mild metabolic acidosis (pH 7.35)
  - Aim for mild hypoventilation (pCO_2 around 60 mmHg)
- In case of pulmonary edema caused by congestion and pulmonary overflow, give intravenous diuretics (1–2 mg/kg furosemide), ensure high PEEP (i.e., 10–15 cm H_2O) and reduce prostaglandin E1 to a minimum (e.g., 10 ng/kg/min)

Note

The administration of oxygen ($SatO_2$ >85%) as a general measure and hyperventilation in children with ductal-dependent systemic circulation can lead to an acute decompensation of the hemodynamic situation.

1.5.2. Cardiac defects with ductal-dependent pulmonary circulation

The situation is reversed in ductal-dependent pulmonary circulation, but the prenatal situation should be achieved too. Again a saturation of 75–85% is adequate and saturations >85% should be avoided as they indicate inadequate pulmonary perfusion. The following measures can be useful to allow more blood to flow from the systemic circulation to the pulmonary circulation via the patent ductus arteriosus if needed:

- Secure patency of the ductus arteriosus via a prostaglandin E1 infusion (initial dosage 20–50 ng/kg/min).
- Lower pulmonary vascular resistance:
  - Aim for mild metabolic alkalosis (use buffering) (pH 7.45–7.5)
  - Adjust ventilation for mild hyperventilation (pCO_2 around 35 mmHg)
  - Increase FiO_2
- Increase systemic vascular resistance and support systemic pressure by:
  - Noradrenaline infusion
  - Possibly also adrenaline infusion
  - Use volume more generously
  - Do not use dopamine
- Maintain rather high dosage of prostaglandin E1.

Excursus: Prostaglandin

Prostaglandin E1 is given to maintain patency or reopen the ductus arteriosus in neonates with ductal-dependent defect. Due to its short half-life, it must be administered continuously intravenous. The initial dosage in a patient with a nearly closed duct is between 50 and 100 ng/kg/min. Based on the actual effect, this dosage can be reduced gradually to a minimum of 5–10 ng/kg/min,

The most common side effects are as follows:

- Apnea (administer in readiness for intubation)
- Bradycadia
- Vasodilatation (pulmonary and systemic), hypotension
- Fever
- Edema
- (Cortical hyperostosis, periostitis only after long-term administration)

Practical tip: When a prostaglandin infusion is required, always a second venous access should be inserted to ensure safe prostaglandin administration immediately via other access if the first one is dislocated. The second access can also be used for volume substitution in case of acute hypotension.

1.5.3. Cardiac defects with parallel circulations

The only example of this cardiac defect is a transposition of the great arteries (d-TGA) together with its variations. The management of this situation is described in the specific treatment section.

1.5.4. Cardiac defects with complete intracardiac mixing of blood

The different cardiac defects (i.e., univentricular hearts) in this group are also described in the following treatment section.

1.5.5. Cardiac defects with a large left-to-right shunt

When the pulmonary resistance drops after the first 4–6 weeks of life, the left-to-right shunt and thereby pulmonary blood flow will increase dramatically. Consequently, heart failure may develop caused by increased volume load, which must be treated medically (diuretics, ACE inhibitors, beta blockers, possibly digoxin or cathecholamines) until corrective surgery is performed. As additional oxygen will lower the pulmonary resistance and increase excessive pulmonary blood flow, no additional oxygen should be administered.

http://dx.doi.org/10.5772/66990

1.6. Specific treatment of the most common symptomatic heart defects in the neonatal period

1.6.1. Left ventricle outflow tract obstruction lesion (i.e., critical aortic stenosis, coarctation of the aorta and interrupted aortic arch)

The initial management of these children has some common features:

- Shock therapy, including intubation and ventilation (high PEEP (>10 cm H_2O) if there is pulmonary edema)
- Prostaglandin E1: initial dosage 50–100 ng/kg/min
- Oxygen: avoid excessive administration, use PEEP to improve oxygenation. (note: oxygen lowers pulmonary resistance and thus increases pulmonary blood flow)
- Use diuretics (furosemide), to manage pulmonary edema and lower preload
- Use catecholamines (dobutamine, adrenaline, NOT dopamine), preferably milrinone depending on blood pressure and myocardial function. (If there is a subvalvular stenosis, catecholamines should be administered with particular caution due to a possible increase in the obstruction.)
- Assess by ECHO and reduce afterload (e.g., sodium nitroprusside)
- Aim for moderate metabolic acidosis (target pH 7.35)
- Administer as little volume as possible; preferably only after cardiac function has recovered or is assessed to be stable in echocardiography

1.6.1.1. Critical aortic stenosis (AoS)

1.6.1.1.1. Hemodynamic situation

Due to the severe obstruction of the aortic valve, the left ventricular function usually is markedly impaired and cannot provide sufficient cardiac output for the systemic circulation which is supplied with blood from the pulmonary artery via the patent ductus arteriosus (i.e., prenatal situation). Left ventricular hypertrophy and possibly fibroelastosis have already developed in utero. This defect is often associated with other left heart obstructions (mitral stenosis, coarctation of the aorta, hypoplastic aortic arch—i.e., Shones complex). If a heart murmur is not already detected in the neonate, many patients with critical aortic stenosis present in severe cardiac shock. In addition, there is differential cyanosis.

In critical AoS with PDA-dependent systemic circulation (prostaglandin infusion), a left-to-right shunt at the atrial level is necessary to allow mixing of the oxygenated pulmonary venous blood via the right atrium, the right ventricle, the pulmonary artery and then the patent ductus arteriosus. A balloon atrial septostomy (Rashkind maneuver) may be necessary, if the shunt at the atrial level is not large enough,

1.6.1.1.2. Further procedure

If suspected ensure prompt transfer to a pediatric cardiac center for interventional catheterization and performance of balloon valvuloplasty (method of choice) or surgical commissurotomy (rarely required); possibly carry out an emergency Rashkind maneuver if there is a restrictive foramen ovale and inadequate left ventricular function after balloon valvuloplasty.

1.6.1.2. Coarctation of the aorta (CoA)

1.6.1.2.1. Hemodynamic situation

In patients with critical CoA, the lower half of the body is supplied with deoxygenated blood from the pulmonary artery via the PDA (differential cyanosis). When the ductus arteriosus closes, dramatic hypoperfusion of the body distal to the aortic isthmus occurs. The left ventricle has now suddenly contract against the pronounced obstruction and rapid decompensation occurs. Associations with other left heart obstructions (bicuspid aortic valve) or a VSD are common.

1.6.1.2.2. Further procedure

Again organize prompt transfer to a pediatric cardiac center for surgical correction, which is generally attempted after the hemodynamic situation has been stabilized. In some special conditions (e.g., for patients in poor general condition or with necrotizing enterocolitis—NEC), primary interventional catheterization with balloon dilatation or implantation of a coronary stent may be indicated for stabilization until surgery.

1.6.1.3. Interrupted aortic arch

1.6.1.3.1. Hemodynamic situation

There are different forms of an interrupted aortic arch and the perfusion of the lower half of the body depends however entirely on a patent ductus arteriosus (i.e., prostaglandin). A VSD is nearly always associated with this defect and other left heart obstructions occur occasionally. Again oxygen saturation should be measured preductally (right hand), as the preductal saturation reflects the situation of the perfusion and blood supply in the CNS and coronary arteries. The levels measured in the lower limbs correspond with pulmonary arterial saturation.

1.6.1.3.2. Further procedure

Prompt transfer to a pediatric cardiac center for surgical correction.

1.6.1.4. Hypoplastic left heart syndrome

1.6.1.4.1. Hemodynamic situation

In patients with a hypoplastic left heart syndrome (HLHS), both the pulmonary and systemic systems are supplied by the right ventricle. Although there are four forms of HLHS (i.e., MA and AoA, MS and AoA, MS and AoS, MA and AoS with VSD), retrograde coronary perfusion takes place in all across the ductus arteriosus with mixed blood from the pulmonary artery and retrogradely across the coarctation and ascending aorta. Within the first few hours of life, the drop in pulmonary resistance together with the manifestation of a coarctation causes the blood from the pulmonary artery to flow primarily into the pulmonary circulation. Therefore, the systemic circulation—together with the coronary arteries—is increasingly less perfused. Severe heart failure develops, which if untreated usually results in shock. As a result, there is severe metabolic acidosis but due to pulmonary recirculation, the oxygen saturation is only moderately reduced. The higher the oxygen saturation is, the more the ratio of pulmonary to systemic perfusion changes are in favor of pulmonary over perfusion and systemic underperfusion. In addition, postnatal closure of the PDA enhances this fatal circulation with underperfusion of the systemic circulation and excessive pulmonary perfusion [9].

It is important to note that oxygenated pulmonary venous blood from the left atrium can only reach the systemic circulation across a sufficiently large shunt to the right atrium (see above).

1.6.1.4.2. Initial treatment

- Shock treatment, including intubation and ventilation (but avoid ventilation if possible, as long as the pH is balanced); hyperventilation must be avoided
- Prostaglandin E1: initial dosage 50–100 ng/kg/min
- Avoid administering oxygen (additionally reduces pulmonary resistance and thus systemic perfusion), target saturation 70–85%
- Administer some furosemide (1–2 mg/kg) to lower preload or for pulmonary edema
- Catecholamine treatment is often required, but should be administered with restraint (can increase the myocardial oxygen consumption), give milrinoneor dobutamine if needed, do not use dopamine
- Possibly reduce afterload (e.g., sodium nitroprusside)
- For severe acidosis, large amounts of NaBic are often required to manage acidosis (doses up to 10 ml/kgbw of NaBic are common!)
- Aim for moderate metabolic acidosis (target pH 7.35, avoid over-buffering)
- As little volume as possible should be administered; preferably only after cardiac function has recovered or is assessed to be stable in echocardiography

1.6.1.4.3. Further procedure

If the atrial defect is restrictive (leading symptom: severe cyanosis, oxygen saturation <65%, seriously ill child), pulmonary congestion has developed and an emergency balloon atrial septostomy (Rashkind maneuver) may be needed.

The patient should be transferred quickly to a pediatric cardiac center for surgery after stabilization (usually a Norwood procedure as the first step of three-stage Fontan palliation).

1.6.2. Right ventricle outflow tract obstruction lesion (critical pulmonary stenosis and pulmonary atresia with intact ventricular septum or ventricular septal defect, tetralogy of fallot, tricuspid atresia with pulmonary stenosis and Ebstein anomaly)

The initial treatment of this group of patients has some common features:

- Prostaglandin E1 infusion: initial dosage 50–100 ng/kg/min
- Initially more generous oxygen therapy (lowers pulmonary resistance)
- Initially more generous volume therapy (i.e., 20 ml/kg bw)
- Try to achieve mild metabolic alkalosis (use over-buffering) (pH 7.45–7.5)
- Possibly ventilation and mild hyperventilation (pCO_2 around 35 mmHg)
- Possibly use an increase in systemic resistance (noradrenaline)

1.6.2.1. Critical pulmonary stenosis

1.6.2.1.1. Hemodynamic situation

A critical pulmonary stenosis is a high-grade obstruction of the pulmonary valve with subsequent hypoxemia. As the right ventricle cannot drain into the pulmonary circulation, secondary hypoxia occurs due to a right-to-left shunt across the foramen ovale/ASD. The musculature of the RV is severely hypertrophic and the RV and tricuspid valve may sometimes be hypoplastic. To ensure oxygenation, the pulmonary circulation is supplied with blood from the aorta via the PDA.

1.6.2.1.2. Further procedure

After diagnosis and prostaglandin infusion organize transfer to a pediatric cardiac center for interventional catheter balloon valvuloplasty.

1.6.2.2. Pulmonary atresia with intact ventricular septum

1.6.2.2.1. Hemodynamic situation

In pulmonary atresia with intact ventricular septum, which can be judged as extreme form of pulmonary stenosis, the right ventricle cannot drain its blood normally to the PA. The majority of blood from the right ventricle either flows back into the right atrium due to tricuspid regurgitation. In addition in some cases, the right ventricle may be connected with the coronary arteries via myocardial sinusoids. In the latter case, the coronary arteries may have other problems and are stenotic so that coronary perfusion may depend on blood flow from the right ventricle (right ventricular dependent coronary circulation (RVDCC). Usually there is suprasystemic pressure in the right ventricle and the right ventricle is hypoplastictic various degrees. Again, the pulmonary circulation is supplied with blood from the aorta via the PDA to ensure oxygenation.

1.6.2.2.2. Further procedure

After stabilization, organize transfer to a pediatric cardiac center. In most cases, cardiac catheterization is needed to rule out myocardial sinusoids and coronary anomalies. In some cases, it is possible to open the right ventricular outflow tract by interventional catheterization or implant a stent into the PDA. Otherwise interim palliative surgery (opening the right ventricular outflow tract or aortopulmonary shunt) must be performed accordingly.

1.6.2.3. Tricuspid atresia

1.6.2.3.1. Hemodynamic situation

In tricuspid atresia, that may give an example for all univentricular heart defects, there is no continuity between the right atrium and ventricle, so the right atrium can drain into the left atrium only across a right-to-left shunt at atrial level. There are various forms of tricuspid atresia depending on the variations of obstructions of the right ventricular outflow tract or pulmonic valve. The RV is usually perfused from the LV across a VSD that is almost always present. The RV is hypoplastic to various extents. Oxygen saturation is identical in the aorta and pulmonary artery because of the complete mixing of blood.

Frequently stenosis and even atresia of the pulmonary artery occur and may have a negative effect on the blood flow to the pulmonary circulation. If there is atresia or a high grade stenosis of the pulmonary artery, perfusion of the lungs depends on a patent ductus arteriosus (see above). In addition, the great vessels can be in normal position or in transposition.

If there is no pulmonary stenosis and blood flow to the pulmonary circulation is unobstructed, the main symptom that may develop later on is heart failure (tachypnea, hepatomegaly, pallor, possible pulmonary edema), but this constellation is much less common.

Initial treatment if there is no pulmonary stenosis (leading symptom: heart failure):

- Anticongestive treatment (diuretics, milrinone, rarely catecholamines)
- Restrictive volume therapy
- Restrictive oxygen therapy

1.6.2.3.2. Further procedure

Transfer to a pediatric cardiac center should be organized. If there is a restrictive atrial shunt (rare), an interventional catheter balloon atrial septostomy (Rashkind maneuver) may be needed. If there is inadequate pulmonary perfusion, a palliative aortopulmonary shunt is placed. The separation of circulations is performed later as multistep procedure (Fontan procedure).

1.6.2.4. Tetralogy of Fallot

1.6.2.4.1. Hemodynamic situation

In tetralogy of Fallot, there is a typical combination of a large VSD with overriding of the aorta, a subpulmonary and pulmonary stenosis, often combined with supravalvular stenosis of various degrees and a marked hypertrophy of the right ventricle. Cyanosis is determined by the extent of the obstruction of the right ventricular outflow tract and thereby pulmonary blood flow. In most cases, this obstruction is only mild at birth, but becomes more significant during the first few weeks of life due to the increase in the infundibular stenosis. If there is pronounced stenosis of the right ventricular outflow tract (functional pulmonary atresia), the children may already develop symptoms with cyanosis or hypoxic spells even in the neonatal period. Hypercyanotic spells occur if there is a sudden increase in subpulmonary muscular obstruction of the RVOT (i.e., agitation) or an acute drop in peripheral vascular resistance (i.e., after feeding).

Treatment of a hypoxic-hypercyanotic spell:

- Immediate sedation (e.g., ketamine IV 2–5 mg/kg, alternatively opiates, benzodiazepines)
- Oxygen therapy
- Increase in systemic resistance by
  - pressing the child's flexed knee against the chest ("jack-knife position")
  - if necessary infusion of vasoconstrictors (noradrenaline)
  - generous volume bolus (e.g., 20–50 ml/kg)
- Compensation of metabolic acidosis by buffering
- Possibly beta blockers (e.g., propranolol IV 0.01–0.1 mg/kg very slowly under monitor guidance)

1.6.2.4.2. Further procedure

Rapid transfer to a pediatric cardiac center is urgently needed. In most circumstances, interventional management can improve the hemodynamic situation (i.e., balloon dilatation of the pulmonary valve, stenting of the right ventricular outflow tract, stenting of a PDA). Only in few cases, early surgical correction is required today. In special situations (e.g., very small children), an aortopulmonary shunt is first placed as a palliative measure to ensure lung perfusion.

1.6.2.5. Pulmonary atresia with ventricular septal defect

1.6.2.5.1. Hemodynamic situation

From the hemodynamic aspect, this disease is an extreme form of Tetralogy of Fallot. Pulmonary perfusion is, however, dependent on a patent ductus arteriosus (prostaglandin infusion) or aortopulmonary collaterals.

1.6.2.5.2. Further procedure

After stabilization with prostaglandin infusion, a rapid transfer to a pediatric cardiac center should be organized. In cases with only membranous valvular atresia, an attempt can be made to open the valve by interventional catheterization (or with stent placement). In addition placing a stent in the PDA may help to achieve catch-up growth of the pulmonary vessels, which are almost always hypoplastic. If this intervention is not possible, an aortopulmonary shunt is placed as surgical palliation. After catch-up growth of the pulmonary vascular system, a continuity between the pulmonary vessels and the right ventricle is created surgically later (e.g., with a valved conduit).

1.6.2.6. Ebstein's anomaly

1.6.2.6.1. Hemodynamic situation

In Ebstein's anomaly, there is apical displacement of the tricuspid valve into the right ventricle combined with moderate to severe tricuspid regurgitation and reduced flow from the small right ventricle to the pulmonary artery. The right atrium is markedly too massively dilated. A pronounced Ebstein's anomaly can already be symptomatic in the neonatal period. Cyanosis occurs due to a right-to-left shunt at the atrial level caused by minimal antegrade flow to the pulmonary artery. In addition, the gross dilatation of the heart may compress the lungs and impair pulmonary function.

The disease may often complicated by accessory pathways (Wolf-Parkinson-White syndrome).

Besides initial treatment stated above, in Ebstein's anomaly:

- If there is heart failure, possibly catecholamines and diuretics
- If there is supraventricular tachycardia, it should be terminated with a vagal maneuver, adenosine, amiodarone, possibly cardioversion

1.6.2.6.2. Further procedure

The goal of surgical treatment is to reconstruct the tricuspid valve and close the ASD. If there is insufficient lung perfusion, it may be necessary to place an aortopulmonary shunt. If there is pronounced hypoplasia of the right ventricle, the univentricular Fontan pathway may be the only option. The overall prognosis is unfavorable for children who become symptomatic already in the neonatal period. These children require urgent transfer to a pediatric cardiac center.

1.6.3. d-transposition of the great arteries (d-TGA)

1.6.3.1. Hemodynamic situation

In d-TGA, there is parallel connection of the pulmonary and systemic circulations; the systemic venous blood is directed back into the aorta and the pulmonary venous blood is pumped back to the pulmonary artery. Survival is only possible if shunts between the two circulatory systems do exist. The most important is a patent foramen ovale or ASD as shunt at atrial level, so oxygenated blood can reach the systemic circulation via the right ventricle across this left-to-right shunt. A PDA has a favorable effect on oxygenation because PDA blood flow increases lung perfusion and as a result the volume load and pressure in the left atrium is increased, so the left-to-right shunt at atrial level increases and more oxygenated blood can reach the systemic circulation [10].

Oxygen application may act indirectly by reducing pulmonary resistance and thus increasing pulmonary perfusion and thereby left atrial volume load and pressure (caution: uncontrolled administration of oxygen can also lead to closure of the ductus arteriosus when used without prostaglandin).

In addition to improve mixing between the two circulations, especially in "poor mixers," an attempt should be made to improve mixed venous saturation.

If there is an associated large VSD, cyanosis is usually less pronounced.

Initial treatment:

- Prostaglandin E1 infusion: initial dosage 50 ng/kg/min
- Generous volume therapy
- Aim for mild metabolic alkalosis (over-buffering) (pH 7.45–7.5, lowers pulmonary resistance)
- Oxygen therapy for severe cyanosis in neonates (caution: induces closure of the ductus arteriosus)
- If possible avoid intubation, ventilation and relaxation (lowers oxygen consumption and therefore increases mixed venous saturation. On the other hand, ventilation increases the intrathoracic pressure, which can impair mixing of the blood)
- Consider the improve cardiac output and thus mixed venous saturation by milrinone
- Generous treatment of anemia (improves oxygen supply)

1.6.3.2. Further procedure

If there is a restrictive shunt at the atrial level, a bedside interventional catheter balloon atrial septostomy (Rashkind maneuver) should be performed as soon as possible before transfer to a pediatric cardiac center. The surgical standard treatment is an arterial switch operation (Jatene procedure) within the first 2 weeks of life.

1.6.4. Truncus arteriosus communis

1.6.4.1. Hemodynamic situation

In a truncus arteriosus communis (TAC), only one vessel (common trunk) arises from the heart. The systemic and pulmonary circulation and the coronaries are here supplied from this

http://dx.doi.org/10.5772/66990

trunk only. A VSD is almost always present. Since the blood follows the path of least resistance and tends to flow into the pulmonary circulation, there is usually excessive pulmonary blood flow after the drop in pulmonary resistance between the second and eighth weeks of life. In this situation, clinical signs of heart failure are already present in the first weeks of life. Due to the significant pulmonary recirculation, there is often only astonishingly mild cyanosis, although the trunk vessel contains only mixed blood.

Initial treatment:

- Oxygen lowers pulmonary resistance and thus increases blood flow to the pulmonary circulation, leading to excessive pulmonary blood flow and increasing heart failure—therefore, use oxygen restrictively
- Treatment of heart failure: diuretics, possibly catecholamines (dobutamine) or phosphodiesterase inhibitor (milrinone), afterload reducer (ACE inhibitor, possibly sodium nitroprusside)
- If associated with an interrupted aortic arch: prostaglandin E1 infusion: initial dosage 50–100 ng/kg/min

1.6.4.2. Further procedure

Organize transfer to a pediatric cardiac center. The definitive correction with a Rastelli procedure is generally performed within the first weeks of life depending on the clinical signs of heart failure.

1.6.5. Total anomalous pulmonary venous connection (TAPVC)

1.6.5.1. Hemodynamic situation

Depending on the location of the anomalous connection of the pulmonary veins, we distinguish between supracardiac, cardiac, infracardiac and mixed forms. Please note that an infracardiac total anomalous pulmonary venous connection is regularly associated with an obstruction at the connection site.

In a total anomalous pulmonary venous connection, all pulmonary veins drain into the systemic venous system and oxygenated blood is guided from there into the right atrium. The perfusion of the systemic circulation thus depends on a right-to-left shunt at the atrial level that is necessary for survival.

In a TAPVC without obstruction of the pulmonary vein, the hemodynamic situation is similar to that of a large ASD (volume overload of the right atrium, ventricle and pulmonary circulation).

Initial treatment:

Total anomalous pulmonary venous connection with obstruction of the pulmonary vein:

- Oxygen therapy
- Intubation and ventilation with a high PEEP (>10 cm H_2O) for pulmonary edema

- Lower PVR: hyperventilation, generous buffering (target pH 7.45–7.5), increase oxygen supply, possibly inhaled NO or prostacyclin IV
- Diuretics, possibly catecholamines for low cardiac output (caution: catecholamines can exacerbate pulmonary edema)

1.6.5.2. Further procedure

A TAPVC with obstruction of the pulmonary vein is an absolute cardiac surgery emergency that must be surgically corrected immediately. Dilatation with or without stent implantation can treat the stenosis of the pulmonary vein in individual cases, so that the surgical repair can be performed after the child is stabilized.

If there is a restrictive atrial shunt or if surgical correction is not possible immediately, an interventional catheter balloon atrial septostomy (Rashkind maneuver) may be considered.

1.6.6. Complete atrioventricular septal defect

1.6.6.1. Hemodynamic situation

In a complete atrioventricular septal defect (AVSD, AV canal), both segments of the ventricular and atrial septum in the region of the AV valves are absent and the development of the AV valves is also impaired. This malformation results in a large left-to-right shunt that increases when the pulmonary resistance drops within the first weeks of life. Children with a complete AVSD usually develop heart failure when the pulmonary resistance drops after 2–8 weeks of life. The situation can be complicated by (mainly systemic) AV valve insufficiency.

Note

trisomy 21 is frequently associated with AVSD. All neonates with trisomy 21 must therefore have an ECHO examination at an early age.

Initial treatment:

- Avoid oxygen (excessive pulmonary blood flow is increased)
- Pharmacological treatment of heart failure: diuretics, ACE inhibitors, beta blockers, rarely catecholamines (possibly digoxin?)

1.6.6.2. Further procedure

The corrective surgery is generally performed at the age of 4–6 months and it may be necessary earlier if conservative heart failure treatment is unsuccessful.

2. Postoperative cardiac intensive care therapy

The following remarks apply primarily to those patients that are transferred immediately after surgery from the surgical operating room and their early postoperative period in the pediatric cardiac intensive care unit (PCICU).

2.1. Basics

One of the main requirements for providing good quality of care in a PCICU is to understand that the job of the intensive care physician starts far before the operated child is admitted to the PCICU. Detailed information on the case of the child is required in advance before the day of admission. The PCICU intensivist must be aware of and understand the hemodynamics of the cardiac defect (i.e., check the ECHO, cath data, etc.), possible complicating or concomitant diseases, the actual planned surgical repair or procedure and the usually possible perioperative and postoperative complications.

Every intensive care physician should be familiar with the major steps of cardiac surgery in general and the specific steps and details of the case to be admitted. These steps include the whole process of surgery from opening the thorax and the mediastinum, thereafter arterial and venous cannulation for the cardiopulmonary bypass, initiation of cardiopulmonary bypass, cardioplegic arrest and finally, the restoration of cardiac function at the end of the operation including decannulation and closure of the thorax.

To obtain this crucial understanding, every intensivist should visit the cardiac theatre on a regular basis and observe about 50 surgeries per year. In complex cases, the intensivist should work together in the time after decannulation or weaning of the bypass with the anesthetist before admission of the patient to the PCICU.

2.2. Preparation of the bed place

The majority of patients will be admitted on a planned and forseeable basis. Before the patient is transferred to the PCICU, a careful and standardized preparation of the bed/place must be completed to avoid unnecessary misunderstanding and streamline the admission process. This preparation may vary from unit to unit but generally includes the following:

- Preparation of the ventilation equipment, adjustment of the settings to the estimated patient-specific parameters, checking of the ventilation bag and mask, oxygen delivery, suction equipment and catheters. In addition, it must be determined by contacting the operating theatre or by assessment of the preoperative information whether iNO (nitric oxide) ventilation is required and possible with the ventilation equipment
- Medication plan: The prepared medication plan should be tailored to the patients' age and weight and include the medication and calculated dosages for the presumed standardized postoperative treatment (i.e., sedation, pain therapy, antibiotics, catecholamines, vasodilators, diuretics, fluid therapy and infusions). The perfusors and flushing solutions should be purged and primed before the patient is transferred to the PCICU

- Monitoring: The bedside monitor is checked beforehand and the patient-specific alarms according to reference values for age and disease are set
- Administrative tasks: Unit specific paperwork is prepared and an X-ray order for the first postoperative X-ray and laboratory order for the first laboratory tests should be prepared

2.3. Postoperative transfer of the patient to the ICU

In order to understand the physiology of the patient, a detailed handover from the different disciplines treating the patient during surgery is necessary. The checklist in **Table 2** contains some common and useful questions that the intensive care physician should discuss with the surgeons, anesthesiologists and cardiac technicians/perfusionists at transfer. The information is crucial and may have direct impact on the subsequent PCICU management.

Surgical aspects
- What were the intraoperative findings? Compared to before?
- What surgical technique was performed? Any problems?
- What drainages were placed intraoperatively (e.g., pleural drainage, mediastinal drainage)?
- What is the assessment of postoperative result?
- Was an intraoperative transesophageal echocardiography performed and what were the findings (residual gradient, valve insufficiency, residual shunt, myocardial function)?
- Did any intraoperative arrhythmias occur? How were they treated?
- Did any intraoperative bleeding problems occur? How were they treated?
Anesthesiology aspects
- Tube size and brand, cuffed and uncuffed?
- Ventilation settings (FiO_2, tidal volume, rate, peak pressure and PEEP)
- Central venous catheter: location of insertion, size
- Arterial access: location, size
- Was an LA or pulmonary artery catheter placed?
- Anesthetics and cardiac medication used (cathecolamines, vasodilators, anti arrhythmics) and their dosages
- Heparinization and current coagulation levels
- Use of blood products (pack red cells, platelet concentrates, fresh frozen plasma)
Cardiopulmonary bypass
- Bypass time
- Aortic cross clamp time
- Cardiac arrest time
- Minimum temperature during bypass
- Was hemofiltration performed at the end of the bypass?

Table 2. Checklist for postoperative transfer.

2.4. Initial examination after transfer to the ICU

Immediately after the patient is admitted to the ICU, the most important clinical parameters must be assessed by the admitting physician and the nurses involved to confirm that the patient is in a stable and safe situation:

- Respiration: Is the chest moving? How are thorax/chest movements? Symmetrical lung expansion? Adequate expansion? How is the Oxygen saturation? FiO2?
- Circulation: Palpation of peripheral pulses (femoral, brachial), visual check of pressure parameters on the monitor (arterial blood pressure, CVP, if inserted pulmonary artery pressure or LA pressure) and check of capillary filling time (normal<2–3 s)
- Diuresis: Is the urine bag filled? How much? Is the bladder filled despite urine catheter? Does the urine look clear or hemolytic? Does the patient appear edematous (puffy) or rather dehydrated?
- Bleeding: Are the drains connected to suction? How much is in the bag and how quick is it filling? Are the secretions dark red (venous blood), bright red (arterial blood), yellowish or clear (serous), warm (fresh) or cold (older)?
- Neurology: is the patient sedated/anesthetized, what is the status of the pupils, are there spontaneous movements and is the patient breathing against the ventilator?
- Body temperature
- Assessment of catheters, lines and cables inserted

During this gross examination to assess the patient's stability, the patient is connected to the bedside monitor system and other equipment. The arterial and central venous accesses are connected with the pressure transducers, set to zero and activated again. The patient is also connected to the ventilator and the drainages set to suction (in general, the suction pressure is set at around 15 cm H_2O). In addition, the external pacemaker is checked for proper function.

In parallel, the first blood samples are taken and include an arterial and central venous blood gas analysis, an ACT and a survey of different pathology markers to asses organ function. The first blood gas analysis including electrolyte status provides information on the ventilation situation, the hemodynamic status (lactate, central venous saturation) and electrolyte metabolism (especially potassium). A standard limb ECG is then recorded, a chest X-ray arranged and finally, an initial exploratory echocardiography (ECHO) performed as a standard in every patient.

2.5. Further postoperative management

2.5.1. Fluid intake

As capillary leak is a normal reaction to bypass and the subsequent inflammatory process induces edema of all organs, the amount of free water intake should be limited postoperatively. Therefore, fluid intake is ideally reduced to 30–50% of the normal maintenance on the first postoperative day and then increased day by day to 75 and finally 100% on the following days.

Patients, however, who underwent cardiac surgery without cardiopulmonary bypass (e.g., resection of an aortic coarctation, PDA ligature) do not require any restriction of postoperative fluid intake.

As soon as the children are able to drink, oral fluid intake should not be restricted any more.

2.5.2. Ventilation

The majority of patients are ventilated after cardiac surgery when they arrive in the PCICU. Pulmonary function is affected by a large variety of preoperative, intraoperative and postoperative factors. Important examples to be considered are listed below:

- Preoperative factors:
  - Preexisting excessive pulmonary blood flow (wet lung, congestion)
  - Preexisting pulmonary hypertension (left-to-right shunt)
  - External compression of the airways, for example, due to vascular rings or prominent pulmonary arteries
- Intraoperative factors:
  - Atelectasis due to surgical manipulation in the thorax or lack of ventilation during the bypass
  - Edema development due to the effect of cardiopulmonary bypass and SIRS
    - Trauma of the lung
- Postoperative factors:
  - Swollen mucosa (SIRS)
  - Atelectasis
  - Lung edema as a result of a postoperative increased lung perfusion. Typical examples are after a shunt procedure or operative opening of circulation in the lungs in pulmonary atresia or severe stenosis ("reperfusion edema")
  - Impaired respiratory mechanics due to postoperative diaphragmatic paresis
  - Pain-related reduction in respiratory capacity (surgery drains)
  - Respiratory depression caused by drugs
  - Pneumothorax, pleural effusions
    - Bleeding through MAPCAS

2.5.3. Settings of the ventilator

Volume-controlled ventilation is the ventilation of choice in every cardiac patient after cardiac surgery. In many ventilators, a setting with a pressure control combination (i.e., PRVC-mode) can be chosen. Hereby markedly, lower rates are usually used (e.g., 20/min for neonates) in the sedated patient. The tidal volume is usually set to 10–15 ml/kg. A relatively long inspiration time is usually selected initially. The PEEP is around 5–10 mmHg and an FiO_2 value is selected at which oxygen saturation of over 95% can be achieved. When the patients waking up, the volume controlled mode is combine with a SIMV mode.

In spontaneous breathing patients, the following values can be used as references for the age-specific respiratory rate:

- Neonates: 40/min
- Infants: 25–30/min
- Toddlers: 25/min
- School-age children: 20/min
- Adolescents: 15/min

Again, in the controlled situation, the rate settings used are much slower.

The following situations are important variants from these initial settings of the ventilator:

- *Univentricular heart*: In univentricular hearts, the balance between systemic and pulmonary circulation is very important to avoid pulmonary overcirculation at the cost of inadequate systemic perfusion. At an oxygen saturation of around 75–85%, a nice balance between systemic and pulmonary perfusion is achieved (Qp/Qs = 1:1). Therefore, the target oxygen saturation in these patients is approximately 80%. Uncritical oxygen administration must be avoided.

- *Fontan circulation*: In these patients, the transpulmonary blood flow is depending completely on the intrathoracic pressure and pulmonary vascular resistance. Theoretically, a high PEEP increases the intrathoracic pressure and thus reduces passive blood across the pulmonary vascular system. A lower PEEP level (<5 mmHg) is therefore often recommended for Fontan patients. On the other hand, a higher PEEP also increases the residual functional capacity and reduces atelectases, so better lung perfusion can be achieved via the Euler–Liljestrand reflex. It has been advocated earlier to ventilate Fontan patients without PEEP—this management strategy is inappropriate and no longer recommended.

- *Pulmonary hypertension*: Pulmonary vascular resistance is reduced by a low pCO_2, a high pH and a high FiO_2. To use this principle, patients with known or presumed pulmonary hypertension (i.e., large VSD, older age, truncus, etc.) should be ventilated using mild hyperventilation (Target pCO_2: 30–35 mmHg) and with higher than normal FiO_2 to achieve an oxygen saturation of around 100% and a paO_2 of more than 150 mmHg

2.5.4. *Infection prophylaxis*

Cardiopulmonary bypass reduces the capacity of the immune system to act against bacterial infections and so postoperative antibiotic prophylaxis is always given for children after cardiac surgery. The antibiotics used and the duration of antibiotic treatment are, however, subject of some controversy. First or second generation cephalosporins are frequently used, for example, cefazolin 30 mg/kg/dose every 8 hourly. For an uncomplicated postoperative course, many centers carry out antibiotic prophylaxis for 2–3 days (6–9 doses, until the drains are out) although hardly any evidence-based data for this procedure are available. For patients with an open sternum or peritoneal dialysis or ECMO, no additional management is required but prolonged treatment is often used in many centers. Antibiotic prophylaxis is then continued for 24 h post-chest closure or ECMO/PD removal.

2.5.5. Sedation

In most centers, a combination of an opiate (morphine, fentanyl) and a benzodiazepine (midazolam) is administered intravenously continuously in the initial postoperative period. Propofol is often used in older children who are sedated for only a short period. No time (2–3 days) or dose (3–8 mg/kg/h) limitation applies in these cases. Lactate levels should be checked on a routine basis.

2.5.6. Analgesia

Surgery itself and the drains in the body after surgery is painful procedure. To reduce postoperative pain, a fixed and standardized combination of non-steroidal analgesics (i.e., paracetamol, ibuprofen) and opiates (morphine, fentanyl) is usually used for analgesia for the first 2–3 days. Patient-controlled analgesia with a PCA pump is also applicable for older children (who can already play a video game).

2.5.7. Kidney function

Kidney function nearly always deteriorates in patients who have undergone cardiac surgery. The use of cardiopulmonary bypass leads to renal impairment and intraoperative fluid loading and inflammatory reactions that result in fluid retention. A negative fluid balance is therefore targeted postoperatively.

Urine excretion reflects a combination of cardiac function and cardiac output in combination with kidney function. In general, a urine excretion of at least 2 ml/kg/h after cardiac surgery is a minimum to ensure adequate fluid balance. Patients most often have a combination of pre-renal kidney failure (low cardiac output, capillary leak, volume deficit) in combination with the direct effects of SIRS on the kidney itself. In addition, a low systemic blood pressure and, in case of ascites, a high intra-abdominal pressure leads to a low perfusion pressure in the kidneys (aggressive drainage of ascites). Other less common examples of renal kidney failure are renal vein thrombosis or iatrogenic kidney damage (aminoglycosides, cyclosporin A). Post-renal kidney failure can be caused by obstructions in the region of the efferent urinary tract (e.g., obstruction of the urinary catheter or the urethra) or simply by increased intra abdominal pressure caused by capillary leak and ascites.

Suitable diuretics in the postoperative phase are primarily loop diuretics (Furosemide, ethacrynic acid). They are administered as a bolus or as a continuous infusion if the response is inadequate. The combination with theophylline sometimes enhances the effect. If excretion is insufficient or the fluid balance is clearly positive, peritoneal fluid drainage, or peritoneal dialysis should be initiated early.

http://dx.doi.org/10.5772/66990

2.6. Common postoperative problems and complications

Typical postoperative problems and their most common causes are summarized in **Table 3**.

Problem	Common causes
Blood pressure too high	Pain, fear, catecholamines, excessive fluid volume, result of the abrupt drug discontinuation (beta blockers, ACE inhibitors); typical postoperative problem after correction of an aortic coarctation. Rare causes: cerebral seizures, hypoglycemia (counter regulation)
Blood pressure too low	Hypovolemia, low cardiac output: limited myocardial function, pericardial effusion, arrhythmia (junctional ectopic tachycardia, AV block), excessive drainage loss, hemorrhage, excessive diuresis; vasodilators, anaphylaxis, sepsis, shock, pneumothorax
Central venous pressure (CVP) too low	Fluid deficit (excessive drainage losses, hemorrhage, excessive diuresis, volume intake too low)
Central venous pressure (CVP) too high	Tense/stiff patient (reaction to wake up, insufficient sedation in ventilation patients); impaired right ventricle function. In patients with univentricular heart, a high CVP suggests poor systemic ventricular or a relevant AV valve regurgitation. Other causes are a pericardial tamponade or pneumothorax
Arterial saturation too low	Atelectasis, hypoventilation, technical problems with the ventilation device, disconnected/ obstructed tube, pneumothorax, pleural effusion, pneumonia, pulmonary edema, pulmonary hemorrhage, secretion, right to left shunt
Arterial saturation too high	In patients with univentricular hearts, saturation over 85% suggest an imbalance between pulmonary and systemic perfusion: excessive blood flow to the lungs and diminished supply to the systemic circulation
Bradycardia	Sinus bradycardia, AV block
Tachycardia	Narrow QRS complexes: sinus tachycardia, supraventricular tachycardia, JET Wide QRS complexes: ventricular tachycardia
Increase in lactate	Poor systemic perfusion, seizures, gut ischemia

Table 3. Typical postoperative problems and the most common causes.

2.6.1. Low cardiac output syndrome (LCOS)

There is a variety of factors that can result in myocardial dysfunction and subsequent low cardiac output postoperatively. Typically, they include an inflammatory reaction to cardiopulmonary bypass, myocardial ischemia and inadequate myocardial function as a result of the intraoperative clamping of the aorta, intraoperative hypothermia, a reperfusion edema, or if a surgical procedure was performed using a ventriculotomy—direct myocardial damage, coronary ischemia, inadequate cardioplegia, mechanical alteration, or an infection.

2.6.1.1. Symptoms

Typical clinical signs of low cardiac output are as follows:

- Tachycardia
- Oliguria

- Delayed capillary filling time (>3–4 s)
- Hypotension
- Decreased pulse pressure
- Reduced mixed venous saturation (Note: a difference between arterial and mixed venous saturation not <20–25% suggests sufficient cardiac output and adequate oxygen supply)
- Metabolic acidosis (BE less than −5)
- High lactate level (>3 mmol/l)

2.6.1.2. Treatment

The treatment of low cardiac output has to focus on the underlying causes which should be eliminated if possible. The following measures depending on the hemodynamic situation are commonly used as follows:

- Volume substitution (in case of hypovolemia)
- Inotropic support (catecholamines (i.e., adrenaline, dobutamine), phosphodiesterase inhibitors, intravenous calcium)
- Afterload reduction (sodium nitroprusside, phosphodiesterase inhibitors)
- Consider hormonal therapy for hypotensive resistance to epinephrine and vasopressors: cortisol for suspected adrenal insufficiency, IV or oral triidothyronine (T3) for euthyroid sick syndrome (low T3 levels with LCOS symptoms)
- Chronotropic support (pacemaker therapy, positive chronotropic drugs)
- Treatment of arrhythmias (amiodarone)
- Ventilation strategy
- Reduction in oxygen consumption (sedation, cooling)
- Mechanical circulatory support (ECMO, LVAD)

2.6.2. Pulmonary hypertensive crisis

Based on the underlying anatomy and pathophysiology, many patients may have a significant elevation of pulmonary pressures or pulmonary vascular resistance before surgery. Typical heart defects for this are those with high flow and pressure driven left-to-right shunt defects (large VSD, AVSD, Truncus, etc.) and those with unrestricted flow over a long period (i.e., >6 or 12 months of age). Postoperatively, there may be a rapid and critical increase in pulmonary arterial pressure or pulmonary vascular resistance in certain situations (i.e., agitation, external stimulation such as suctioning, pain, etc.). The result of a rapid increase in PVR is a standstill of the trans-pulmonary blood flow with secondary congestion in the right atrium (high CVP) and ventricle and drop in pressure in the left atrium and ventricle (low CO and BP). Ultimately, cardiac output collapses and the coronaries are not perfused. The following patients are at a particularly high risk for this type of crisis:

http://dx.doi.org/10.5772/66990

- Patients with already increased pulmonary vascular resistance preoperatively (primary pulmonary hypertension)
- Neonates within the first week of life
- Patients with pulmonary venous hypertension (e.g., within the context of a total anomalous pulmonary venous connection or mitral stenosis)
- Older children with a still uncorrected high flow and pressure shunt defects that led to an increase in pulmonary vascular resistance (e.g., complete AV canal, large VSD, truncus)

The following factors may increase pulmonary vascular resistance:

- Hypoxia
- Acidosis (pH <7.3, BE less than −5)
- High partial pressure of carbon dioxide ($paCO_2$ >50)
- Polycythemia
- Atelectasis
- Agitation

The following factors may reduce pulmonary vascular resistance:

- Oxygen administration
- Alkalosis
- Hyperventilation
- NO inhalation (nitric oxide)
- Recruitment of atelectatic lung segments

Prophylaxis of a pulmonary hypertensive crisis is crucial, the acute management as well as the prophylaxis of a pulmonary hypertensive crisis includes the following measures:

- Sufficient analgesia and sedation or relaxation for 1–2 days
- Oxygenation (paO_2 >150)
- Optimizing the ventilation (adequate PEEP)
- Slightly alkalotic pH level (target pH 7.4–7.5) and mild hyperventilation ($paCo_2$ 30–35)
- Pharmacological vasodilators (NO, iloprost, prostacyclin)
- Avoidance of unnecessary manipulations such as too frequent suctioning

2.7. Specific early postoperative problems

Cardiac defects or surgery-specific postoperative problems and complications are summarized in **Table 4**.

Cardiac defect/operation	Specific early postoperative problems and complications
ASD closure	Sinus node dysfunction, left heart failure/pulmonary edema in older children and adults
VSD closure	Pulmonary hypertensive crisis, complete AV block, JET, residual shunt
AV canal correction	Pulmonary hypertensive crisis, complete AV block, JET, AV valve stenosis or incompetence
PDA ligation	Injury to the recurrent laryngeal nerve (vocal cord paralysis) or the thoracic duct (chylothorax), accidental ligation or injury to surrounding vessels (especially left pulmonary artery, aorta
Truncus arterious correction	Pulmonary hypertensive crisis, truncus valve stenosis or incompetence, right ventricular dysfunction
Aortopulmonary window (correction)	Pulmonary hypertensive crisis, coronary ischemia
Anomalous pulmonary venous connection (correction)	Pulmonary hypertensive crisis, atrial arrhythmia, residual stenosis of the pulmonary veins or pulmonary vein anastomosis with the left ventricle, high left ventricular filling pressure due to the relatively small left atrium and ventricle
Fallot correction	Right ventricular diastolic dysfunction (poor compliance of the hypertrophic ventricle), JET, complete AV block, residual pulmonary stenosis, residual VSD, pulmonary insufficiency after a transannular patch
Pulmonary atresia with intact ventricular septum	Right ventricular dysfunction, myocardial ischemia due to right ventricle dependent coronary circulation, circular shunting due to creation of an aortopulmonary shunt and opening of right ventricular outflow tract
Aortic stenosis correction	Residual stenosis, disruption of left ventricular diastolic function, aortic insufficiency, AV block
Ross procedure	Coronary ischemia
Konno procedure	Coronary ischemia, obstruction of the right ventricular outflow tract, arrhythmias (e.g., AV block), mitral regurgitation
Subaortic stenosis (resection)	Residual stenosis, mitral valve injury, (ventricular) arrhythmia, AV block
Coarctation of the aorta (resection)	Residual obstruction, paraplegia, post-coarctectomy syndrome, unmasking an aortic valve stenosis, injury to the recurrent laryngeal nerve, chylothorax
Interrupted aortic arch (correction)	Residual obstruction, compression of the left main bronchus by the aorta, injury to the recurrent laryngeal nerve, chylothorax
Mitral stenosis correction	Pulmonary hypertensive crisis, residual stenosis, mitral regurgitation, left ventricular dysfunction
Creation of an aortopulmonary shunt	Imbalance between systemic and pulmonary perfusion, shunt leak, shunt thrombosis, pulmonary edema, coronary ischemia
Pulmonary artery banding	Cyanosis, insufficient banding (excessive pulmonary blood flow), Qp-Qs mismatch
Norwood procedure	Low cardiac output, imbalance between systemic and pulmonary perfusion, residual obstruction of the aortic arch, AV valve insufficiency, SIRS
Superior cavopulmonary anastomosis (Glenn, Hemifontan)	Cyanosis, hypertension, edema/congestion of the upper half of the body, Chylothorax
Fontan completion	Ascites, pleural effusions, edema, cyanosis, low cardiac output, arrhythmias

http://dx.doi.org/10.5772/66990

Cardiac defect/operation	Specific early postoperative problems and complications
TGA (switch operation)	Coronary ischemia, left ventricular dysfunction, neo aortic insufficiency, peripheral pulmonary stenosis
TGA (Mustard/Senning atrial baffle procedure)	Pulmonary or systemic venous obstruction, atrial arrhythmias
Bland-White-Garland syndrome (correction)	Myocardial dysfunction, mitral regurgitation

Table 4. Specific early postoperative problem and complications (modified from Schwartz and Millar 2009 in Roger's Handbook of Pediatric Intensive care).

2.8. Postoperative features of heart defects with a univentricular heart

The large group of heart defects with a univentricular physiology may pose great challenges to postoperative intensive care in the PCICU. These patients include those with a hypoplastic left heart syndrome, tricuspid atresia, or a double inlet left ventricle. The most important principles in the postoperative treatment of these patients are presented below. As an example, the three-stage surgical procedure for patient with a hypoplastic left heart syndrome is explained. In general, palliation in a Fontan procedure is made with the goal of achieving complete separation of the pulmonary and systemic circulation to eliminate cyanosis. The lungs are perfused passively from the vena cavae without any pumping chamber in between. The single ventricle supplies only the systemic circulation and thereby has a reduced volume load.

The three stages are as follows:

- Norwood procedure or Damus-Kaye-Stansel procedure with a shunt
- Upper cavopulmonary anastomosis (Glenn procedure, "hemi Fontan")
- Total cavopulmonary anastomosis (Fontan procedure)

2.8.1. Norwood procedure

The Norwood procedure is the first step for patients with a hypoplastic left heart syndrome toward separation of the circulatory systems by a Fontan procedure. There are several modifications of this surgical procedure (classical Norwood, Norwood-Sano-procedure). The principal goal is to form a neo-aorta from the pulmonary artery and the hypoplastic aorta that can supply the systemic circulation with blood without a pressure gradient (i.e., unobstructed systemic blood flow). To achieve this, the pulmonary artery and the hypoplastic aorta are anastomosed distal to the valves. Additional patch material is usually required for the reconstruction of the aortic arch and excision of the coarctation. In this manner, a strong vessel for systemic perfusion is created. The pulmonary artery is transected shortly before the pulmonary artery bifurcation and in most cases, pulmonary perfusion is ensured via an aortopulmonary shunt or Sano shunt (placement of a conduit through right ventricular to pulmonary artery).

To achieve the unobstructed inflow to the heart and outflow from the pulmonary veins, an atrial septectomy is also performed. There is a balance between the pulmonary and systemic circulatory systems when arterial saturation is between 75 and 85% (Qp/Qs = 1).

Typical problems after a Norwood procedure are low cardiac output, capillary leak caused by SIRS and hypoxemia.

2.8.1.1. Low cardiac output

As a typical result of the long bypass time required or even prolonged circulatory arrest, a systemic inflammatory response syndrome (SIRS) of various degrees occurs in these neonates. As a consequence, myocardial function is usually markedly impaired so that a certain and often higher amount of catecholamine support is always needed postoperatively. Other possible causes of inadequate systemic perfusion are increased pulmonary perfusion at the expense of systemic perfusion (Qp/Qs >1; leading symptoms: arterial saturation>85%, tachycardia, hypotension, oliguria, metabolic acidosis). To manage this situation, an attempt is made by reducing the afterload of the systemic circulation and increasing pulmonary resistance. AV valve insufficiency or arrhythmias can also cause or deteriorate low cardiac output.

2.8.1.2. Hypoxemia

Hypoxemia (i.e., saturation <70%) can be the result of an imbalance between pulmonary and systemic circulations to the detriment of the pulmonary circulation—for example, in an obstruction of the aortopulmonary shunt or increased pulmonary resistance.

Other causes are typical pulmonary problems such as atelectasis, a pleural effusion, edema, or pneumonia. Peripheral cyanosis occurs with low cardiac output or increased oxygen consumption (leading symptom: reduced systemic venous saturation).

2.8.2. Superior cavopulmonary anastomosis

The aim of a superior cavopulmonary anastomosis is to allow passive blood flow from the upper half of the body into the pulmonary circulation. The superior vena cava is anastomosed in an end-to side manor with the pulmonary artery and thereby the systemic venous blood from the upper half of the body then flows passively to the lungs without an intermediate pumping chamber and is oxygenated there. The systemic venous blood from the lower half of the body does not reach the lungs, but is mixed with the pulmonary venous blood in the heart and pumped into the systemic circulation. The systemic circulation thus contains mixed blood. The saturation of these children is usually about 80–85%.

This step leads to a complete hemodynamic unloading of the univentricular heart as the pulmonary circulation and systemic circulation are now connected in series. The Qp/Qs ratio is then 0.6–0.7; oxygen saturation is 80–85%. In comparison with older children, the head and upper limbs in young children are relatively large and therefore, the overall ratio of pulmonary perfusion is still higher in younger children. The percentage of systemic venous blood

http://dx.doi.org/10.5772/66990

from the upper half of the body, that reaches the lungs via the cavopulmonary anastomosis and is oxygenated there, is correspondingly higher.

Typical postoperative problems are increased pressure in the superior vena cava, hypertension and hypoxemia.

2.8.2.1. *Elevated pressure in the superior vena cava*

In a superior cavopulmonary anastomosis, elevated pressure in the superior vena cava suggests an obstruction in the area of the cavopulmonary anastomosis or pulmonary circulation or elevated pulmonary vascular resistance.

The difference in pressure between the superior vena cava and atrium (transpulmonary gradient) should be <10 mmHg. A high pressure in the superior vena cava can restrict cerebral outflow and lead to marked edema in the upper half of the body (superior vena cava syndrome).

After this operation, patients should be positioned with the upper body elevated (about 45°, half sitting position). Elevated intrathoracic pressure from mechanical ventilation additionally hinders passive blood flow from the superior vena cava into the pulmonary circulation and patients should therefore be quickly extubated.

2.8.2.2. *Hypertension*

Temporary hypertension during the first few postoperative days is not unusual in these patients. The elevation of intracranial pressure that is necessary to maintain adequate cerebral perfusion pressure may be one reason. Aggressive lowering of the blood pressure should therefore be avoided but normal arterial pressures should be obtained.

2.8.2.3. *Hypoxemia*

Saturation levels below 75% following a superior cavopulmonary anastomosis can be caused by many reasons all resulting in a reduction in pulmonary perfusion. This may be due to an obstruction in the area of the anastomosis or pulmonary vessels. Another possible explanation is that blood from the upper half of the body is conducted past the alveoli, for example, if there are venovenous collaterals (connections between the systemic and pulmonary veins), the azygos vein was not ligated by the surgeon, a left sided superior vena cava has reopened or arteriovenous collaterals (connections between the pulmonary arteries and veins) have gained importance.

In the early postoperative phase, arterial saturation can often be improved by attempting mild hypoventilation. Slightly elevated pCO_2 (>50 mmHg) causes vasodilatation of the cerebral vessels, so more blood flows to the brain. Since this allows relatively more blood to reach the upper half of the body, more blood is conducted through the SVC and into the lungs and becomes oxygenated. In addition, the blood can also be slightly alkalized by administering sodium bicarbonate (target pH >7.4).

2.8.3. *Total cavopulmonary anastomosis (Fontan procedure)*

In a Fontan procedure (total cavopulmonary anastomosis), the pulmonary and systemic circulation are finally completely separated by anastomosing the inferior vena cava also with the pulmonary circulation. A tunnel is created that connects the inferior vena cava with the pulmonary artery. This tunnel may pass either through the atrium (intracardiac Fontan) or alternatively outside the heart (extracardiac tunnel). It should be standard to leave a small shunt between the Fontan tunnel and the atrium (i.e., Fontan fenestration) that functions as an overflow (right-to-left shunt) if the resistance in the pulmonary circulation is too high and not all of the systemic venous blood can enter the pulmonary circulation. This may have the disadvantage of mild hypoxemia but the positive effects (improved systemic circulation, decompression of the venous side, less ascites, edema, etc.) clearly overweigh the disadvantage of lower saturations.

When the Fontan circulation is completed, all of the systemic venous blood (exception: coronary sinus) flows passively into the pulmonary circulation without passing through a pumping ventricle. The oxygenated blood is then pumped into the systemic circulation by the univentricular heart.

Typical postoperative problems are low cardiac output, hypoxemia, effusions, arrhythmias and thrombosis.

2.8.3.1. *Low cardiac output*

In Fontan patients, low cardiac output can often occur due to low preload (hypovolemia), increased pulmonary resistance, or an obstruction in the area of the systemic venous outflow (tunnel stenosis, anastomosis stenosis). Therefore, higher volume requirements are often necessary in these patients. In addition, poor ventricular function or AV valve insufficiency and arrhythmias can also cause low cardiac output.

2.8.3.2. *Arrhythmias*

As the completion of the Fontan procedure require surgical manipulation at the atrium and the area of the sinus node, atrial arrhythmias may occur and sinus node dysfunction is typical. A pacemaker (atrial stimulation) sometimes becomes necessary.

2.8.3.3. *Hypoxemia*

Cyanosis can be the result of a relevant right-to-left shunt across a tunnel fenestration. In addition, the usual pulmonary problems (i.e., pleural effusion, atelectasis, pneumonia) can also lead to hypoxemia. Reduced pulmonary perfusion, caused by arteriovenous or venovenous collaterals can also cause hypoxemia in Fontan patients.

2.8.3.4. *Effusions*

Pleural effusions and ascites are common immediately after surgery. They can be the result of elevated venous pressure and volume load required and may lead to considerable postoperative complications.

2.8.3.5. Thrombosis

Based on the low flow in the Fontan circuit, these patients are at an increased risk of developing venous thrombosis. This risk is increased especially if there is low cardiac output. Most centers therefore recommend lifelong anticoagulation for Fontan patients. There is, however, no uniform opinion with respect to the duration or the form of anticoagulation (vitamin K antagonists or platelet aggregation inhibitors). While many different anticoagulation regimens are used in small children (no anticoagulation, aspirin, warfarin), there is a general consensus that anti-coagulation is obligatory in patients after puberty.

Acknowledgements

Parts of this book chapter are similar to a recent publication of the third author [11]. Based on the content of the scientific information, this is, however, current state-of-the-art knowledge and medical management; therefore, similarities in the text are logical necessity.

Author details

Eva Miranda Marwali[1]*, Beatrice Heineking[2] and Nikolaus A. Haas[2]

*Address all correspondence to: evamarwali@yahoo.com

1 Pediatric Cardiac Intensive Care Unit, National Cardiovascular Center Harapan Kita, Jakarta, Indonesia

2 Department of Pediatric Cardiology and Pediatric Intensive Care Medicine, University Hospital of Munich, Ludwig Maxmilians University, Munich, Germany

References

[1] Allen HD, et al. Moss and Adams' heart disease in infants, children and adolescents including the fetus and young adult. Philadelphia: Lippincott Williams & Wilkins; 2008.

[2] Chang AC, et al. Pediatric cardiac intensive care. Philadelphia: Lippincott Williams & Wilkins; 1998.

[3] Cloherty JP, Eichenwald EC, Stark AR. Manual of neonatal care. Philadelphia: Lippincott Williams & Wilkins; 2008.

[4] Driscoll DJ. Fundamentals of pediatric cardiology. Philadelphia: Lippincott Williams & Wilkins; 2006.

[5] Helfaer MA, Nichols DG. Roger's handbook of pediatric intensive care. Philadelphia: Lippincott Williams & Wilkins; 2009.

[6] Keane JF, Lock JE, Fyler DC. Nadas' pediatric cardiology. Philadelphia: Saunders Elsevier; 2006.

[7] Kretz FJ, Becke K. Anesthesia and Pediatric Intensive Care Medicine. Stuttgart: Thieme; 2007.

[8] Park MK. Pediatric cardiology for practitioners. Philadelphia: Mosby Elsevier; 2008.

[9] Alsoufi B, Bennetts J, Verma S, Caldarone CA. New developments in the treatment of hypoplastic left heart syndrome. Pediatrics 2007;119:109–117.

[10] Derrick G, Cullen S. Transposition of the great arteries. Curr Treat Options Cardiovasc Med 2000;2:499–506.

[11] Haas NA, Kleideiter U. Pediatric cardiology—symptoms, diagnosis—treatment. Stuttgart, New York, Delhi, Rio de Janeiro: Thieme Verlag; 2015.

Section 5

Management of Caustic Ingestion in Children

Chapter 6

Caustic Ingestion

Abdulkerim Temiz

Additional information is available at the end of the chapter

http://dx.doi.org/10.5772/67526

Abstract

Caustic ingestion with resultant esophagitis and gastritis is still an important social and medical problem due to early and long-term complications. This injury is seen frequently as an accidental event and may also lead to psychosocial impacts, including antisocial behavior, suicide attempts, criminal incarceration, and educational delinquency. It often occurs as a result of uncontrolled and unsafe storage of materials used in household cleaning. Despite the various treatment proposals, optimal management of the patients remains controversial. The presentation of the depth and extent of injury with endoscopy plays a key role in treatment planning. In the absence of life-threatening complications, the general approach is conservative management in the acute period. The most common complications are esophageal stricture and gastric outlet obstruction. Different treatment methods such as bougienage, stent application, balloon dilation, or esophageal replacement are used in the treatment of the caustic esophageal strictures. The decision of the least invasive method for the treatment of complications will reduce the potential hazardous results.

Keywords: caustic, esophagitis, esophageal stenosis, pyloric stenosis

1. Introduction

Caustic ingestion, which can cause severe morbidity and mortality, is still an important problem worldwide, especially in developing countries, which have an uncontrolled market selling cheap cleaning solutions of unknown composition. Despite several educational and public health initiatives to prevent caustic ingestion in children, in the United States (US), an estimated 5000–15,000 cases of caustic ingestion (incidence 1.08 per 100,000) occur each year [1]. Caustic ingestion also imposes a severe economic burden in terms of medical costs, as children with caustic injuries incurred hospital charges greater than $22 million US dollars in 2009. It is thought that the total costs exceed these amounts when indirect costs such as parental lost income or lodging for parents during hospitalization of children are factored in. These injuries may also lead to psychosocial impacts, including antisocial behavior, suicide attempts, criminal incarceration, and educational delinquency, as well as domestic problems such as family break-up, relocation, or loss of employment. De Jong et al. reported that 50% of children who ingested a caustic substance developed behavioral or educational problems [2]. Moreover, 25% of the families of severely affected children developed domestic problems [2]. Caustic injury may occur via accidental ingestion or as a suicide attempt. Caustic injury is usually more serious inpatients who attempted suicide as compared with accidental ingestion [3]. These cases usually occur in low income and poorly educated families [4]. The age distribution of caustic injury shows a bimodal pattern [1]. The first peak is seen in children between 1 and 5 years of age. In this period, injuries always occur due to accidental ingestion. De Jong et al. reported caustic injured patients aged as young as 1 month [2]. This usually occurs due to incorrect preparation of baby food with a liquid caustic substance accidentally in infancy or the neonatal period [2, 5]. The second peak of distribution is seen during and after the pubertal period; the majority of the cases are suicide attempts [6]. The type of ingested substances varies by geography. While alkaline ingestion is usually seen in more developed countries, acidic ingestion is seen usually in developing countries.

2. Etiology and pathophysiology

Caustic ingestion often occurs as a result of uncontrolled and unsafe storage of materials used in household cleaning. The extent and outcome of caustic ingestion depends on the identity of the caustic substance, as well as the concentration, the pH, the duration of contact between the substance and tissue, and the physical form of the substance. Increased free oxygen radical production, which arises due to ischemia and direct injury, leads to excessive tissue damage in addition to direct injury from the substance. Increased tissue or blood levels of free oxygen radicals have been demonstrated in different experimental studies [7–9]. Ischemic injury occurs during the first 1–4 days, which is defined as the acute necrotic phase. Severe inflammation, necrosis, edema, and hemorrhage are observed during this period. The second period is the subacute phase, usually observed between 4 and 15 days of injury. Mucosal sloughing, bacterial invasion, mucosal ulcer with fibrin crusts and increased granulation tissue due to fibroplasia and increased collagen deposition are the main findings in the second period. Because the aforementioned healing tissue is quite fragile, esophageal perforation or complications of endoscopy may occur during this period. Thus, endoscopy is only recommended in the first 24–48 hours or 2 weeks after the injury. The chronic or cicatrization phase begins at the end of the second week and may continue for several months.

The majority of reported cases are alkaline ingestions. Alkaline ingestion causes liquefaction necrosis, saponification of fats, penetration into the deeper layers, denaturation of proteins, emulsification of cellular membranes, and thrombosis of blood vessels [10]. Because of the greater viscosity of alkaline substances compared to acidic substances, prolonged contact with the substance often occurs in alkaline ingestion. Traditionally, alkaline substances cause tissue damage at pH levels higher than 11.5. It has been reported that a 30% solution of sodium

http://dx.doi.org/10.5772/67526

hydroxide is able to induce a full thickness injury in 1 second. Additionally, caustic injury may occur with a lower concentration but a longer contact time. Mattos et al. demonstrated that the level of macroscopic and microscopic injury mainly depends on the concentration used as the aggressiveness of injuries gradually increases. Even a caustic soda solution at a concentration of 1.83% is able to induce epithelial necrosis in 1 hour [11]. However, they concluded that solution concentration revealed to be most important determinant in injury. Acidic injury causes coagulation necrosis; this results in the formation of an eschar, which limits the depth of penetration and injury. Injury related to acidic ingestion usually occurs with substances with a pH <2. Because of protective effects of eschar formation and rapid transit to the stomach due to low viscosity, acidic ingestion results in more gastric injury than alkaline ingestion. Commonly, gastric injury and complications occur in patients who have ingested an acidic substance, while alkaline ingestion is associated with esophageal injury and complications. Although Temiz et al. diagnosed severe gastric injury in 40.27% of acid-ingesting patients and in 10.71% of alkaline-ingesting patients, there was no difference in the rate of esophageal stricture development between these patients [5]. However, Ciftci et al. reported that the gastric outlet obstruction rate is higher with alkaline ingestion than acidic ingestion [12].

Caustic ingestion may also cause airway injury, resulting in laryngeal and lower airway edema and respiratory distress [5, 6]. Additionally, fibroblast proliferation occurs as a result of caustic injury due to alkaline or acid ingestion, resulting in circular and longitudinal contraction in the submucosal and muscular layers. The clinical manifestations are esophageal stricture, gastric outlet obstruction, gastroesophageal reflux, and hiatal hernia [10].

3. Clinical presentation

Caustic ingestion is seen frequently as an accidental event in children, especially in low income families. It usually occurs between 1 and 3 years of age [2]. The male/female ratio shows a male predominance. Clinical presentations of caustic ingestion vary from no injury to fatal complications. The outcomes and clinical findings depend on the properties of the caustic substance such as type, amount, physical form and depth, and extent of injury. Solid substances may adhere to the mucosa and be difficult to swallow. Therefore, solid substances commonly cause upper level damage, such as upper respiratory, oral cavity, or pharynx injury. Liquid substances may be swallowed easily. Thus, injury to the lower levels such as the esophagus or the stomach occurs more frequently with liquid substances. In the early stage, patients may refer with vomiting, excessive salivation, refusal to drink, apparent oral mucosal findings that vary from mild hyperemia to severe edema and diffuse fibrin sheets on lips, oral, or oropharyngeal mucosa [5, 13, 14]. Respiratory distress, stridor, hoarseness, aphonia, and dyspnea indicate respiratory tract injury. Drooling, dysphagia, odynophagia, and chest or abdominal pain usually observed in severely injured patients. Nausea or hematemesis also may occur. Gaudreault et al. reported severe esophageal burns in only 18–33% of patients with specific clinical signs and symptoms of caustic injury [13]. They concluded that positive clinical signs or symptoms cannot predict esophageal injury. Although they recommended endoscopic evaluation in symptomatic patients, they did not suggest endoscopy for asymptomatic patients, especially those with a questionable history [13]. Temiz et al. reported severe esophageal injury in 19.3% of patients with no symptoms whereas nearly 60% of their patients with significant physical findings had no or mild esophageal injury [5]. Boskovic and Stankovic reported that 6.03% of patients with normal clinical findings had severe esophageal injuries, whereas 66.6% of patients with positive clinical findings had no or mild esophageal findings [15]. Additionally, severe gastric injury was seen in 6.8% of caustic ingestion patients; 1.7% of them had no clinical signs whereas 5.1% of them had positive clinical findings. These results show that the sensitivity and specificity of clinical findings regarding esophageal injury are 74 and 73%, respectively, with a positive predictive value of 0.33 and a negative predictive value of 0.66. They calculated these values as sensitivity 75%, specificity 68%, positive predictive value 0.15, and negative predictive value 0.97 for gastric injury [15]. Temiz et al. observed severe gastric injury in 18.5% of all caustic ingestion patients; 3.9% of these patients had normal physical findings whereas 14.6% of them had positive clinical findings [5]. Fifty percent of patients who developed gastric outlet obstruction did not have physical findings [5]. They calculated the sensitivity and specificity of clinical findings regarding severe esophageal injury as 80.6 and 32.8%, respectively. Also, they reported the sensitivity and specificity of clinical findings regarding severe gastric injury as 75.7 and 29%, respectively. Severe complications, including severe esophageal or gastric injury (especially transmural necrosis or perforation), should be considered in patients with abdominal/chest pain and hematemesis. More serious and fatal presentations secondary to caustic ingestion, such as disseminate intravascular coagulation, tracheoesophageal fistula, brachiocephalic fistula, paralyzed vocal cords, and acute pancreatitis have been reported [16, 17].

Button battery ingestion seems to cause the most severe injuries. Button battery tends to become lodged at areas of physiological narrowing in the gastrointestinal tract, such as the pharyngoesophageal junction, gastroesophageal junction, pylorus, ligament of Treitz, Meckel diverticulum or ileocecal valve (**Figure 1a** and **b**). Larger batteries usually tend to be affixed in the esophagus, whereas smaller batteries pass into the stomach and intestine [18]. Especially, button batteries with a diameter of 20 mm or larger can become lodged in the esophagus in children [19]. The complications associated with button battery ingestion are the result of a combination of four mechanisms, including leakage of the alkaline substance, absorption of the toxic substance, and necrosis secondary to either direct pressure from the battery or electrical discharge [18]. Votteler et al. demonstrated that mucosal necrosis occurred within 1 hour and ulceration within 2 hours of battery placement in an experimental study [20]. Litovitz et al. reported that batteries become lodged within 4 hours of ingestion, and esophageal perforation occurs 6 hours after ingestion [21]. These results are related to the site at which the battery is lodged, the contact time and the possibility of heavy metal absorption [18, 20, 22]. The complications of esophageal impactions are more severe than those of lower gastrointestinal impactions. The most dangerous complications, such as esophageal or aortic perforation, trachea-esophageal fistula, hemorrhagic shock, severe esophageal bleeding, and vocal cord paralysis, have been observed in patients with esophageal button battery impactions [19]. Fatal aorto esophageal fistula and perforation of the brachiocephalic artery secondary to button battery ingestion have been reported in children [23, 24].

The clinical complaints of late presenting patients are slightly different. Generally, after 3 weeks, the patients may admit with dysphagia, vomiting, or respiratory problems [25]. These complaints

http://dx.doi.org/10.5772/67526

(a) (b)

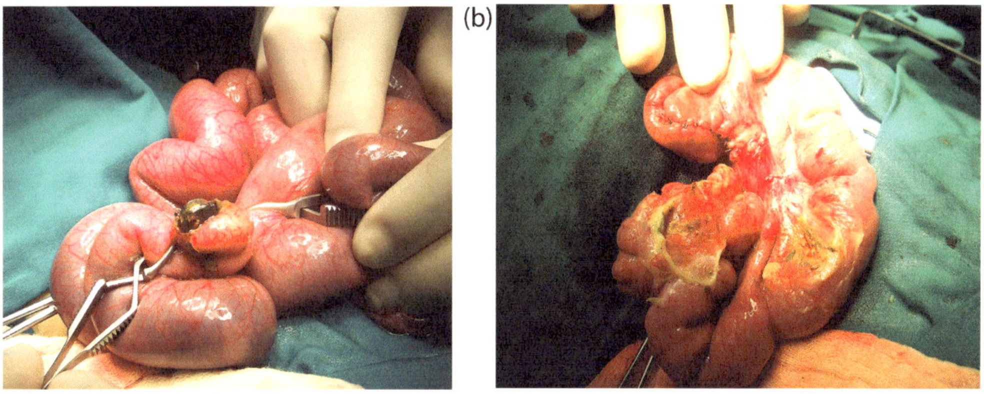

Figure 1. Perforation of Meckel's diverticulum by button battery (a) and caustic injury of adjacent intestinal segments (b).

indicate late complications such as esophageal stricture, gastric outlet obstruction, or gastroesophageal reflux. Late complications especially esophageal strictures or gastric outlet obstructions cause dysphagia, insufficient oral intake or vomiting. Malnutrition, growth retardation, feeding intolerance, dehydration or liquid and electrolyte imbalance may develop secondary to these symptoms and complications. Obstructive complications usually occur at the level of physiological narrowing of the gastrointestinal tract, especially at three esophageal narrowing and the pylorus.

3.1. Staging

Staging is important to separate severely injured patients from mildly injured or healthy children. The classification of patients allows for the identification of patients at risk of developing early or late complications. Several different grading systems have been described and suggested in previous studies [26, 27]. The modification of the method of Di Costanzo grading system is summarized in **Table 1** [5, 28]. All classifications based on endoscopic findings have been prepared on the basis of mucosal findings, mucosal involvement, and the depth of injury.

Grade	Findings
0	Normal
1	Mucosal edema Hyperemia
2a	Hemorrhagic mucosa Bullous mucosa Exudates Fibrinous membranes Superficial ulceration
2b	Circumferential ulceration (addition to the grade 2a)
3	Scattered small necrotic area Hemorrhagic black or brown mucosa

Table 1. Modify Di Costanzo classification [5, 28].

Most researchers make modifications to previously described grading systems [3, 28]. The most preferred staging systems were Di Costanzo and Zargar grading system or their modifications [3, 10, 26–29]. Additionally, Ryu et al. have described a classification according to computed tomography findings. Computed tomography has been suggested to be more effective for the evaluation of transmural injuries to esophagus and stomach as well as necrosis [30, 31]. In our opinion, this type of imaging is advantageous in selected cases, especially in patients with necrosis or perforation, although the radiation effects of computed tomography must be considered.

3.2. Complications

The complications that develop secondary to caustic ingestion are divided into early and long-term complications. Early complications are usually related to the acute effects of the caustic substance, which generally manifest as tissue necrosis. Chemical pneumonitis, atelectasis, aspiration pneumonia, and dysphagia are some of early complications due to the acute effects of ingestion [2]. Tracheoesophageal fistula is another early stage complication. Poley et al. detected severe systemic complications more frequently among patients who ingested acidic substances than those who drank alkaline substances in their report on adolescent and adult patients [28]. They reported renal insufficiently, hepatic dysfunction, diffuse intravascular coagulation, and hemolysis as systemic complications [28]. These authors reported 16% overall mortality. They showed a worse death rate with the ingestion of acidic substances compared with alkaline substances (14 vs. 2%); 11% of overall mortality was related to systemic complications [28]. Early complications may also have catastrophic consequences, and some complications can result in death [23]. Ulceration, edema, gastrointestinal hemorrhage, total loss of the vocal cord, vocal cord paresis, denuded epiglottis, aorta esophageal fistula, esophageal perforation, perforation of Meckel's diverticulum, and perforation of the brachiocephalic artery are early stage complications that have been reported previously [18, 19, 24, 32–37]. Acute pancreatitis has been reported as an early complication secondary to accidental caustic ingestion in a young adult [16]. Skin injuries are seen in some cases (**Figure 2a** and **b**).

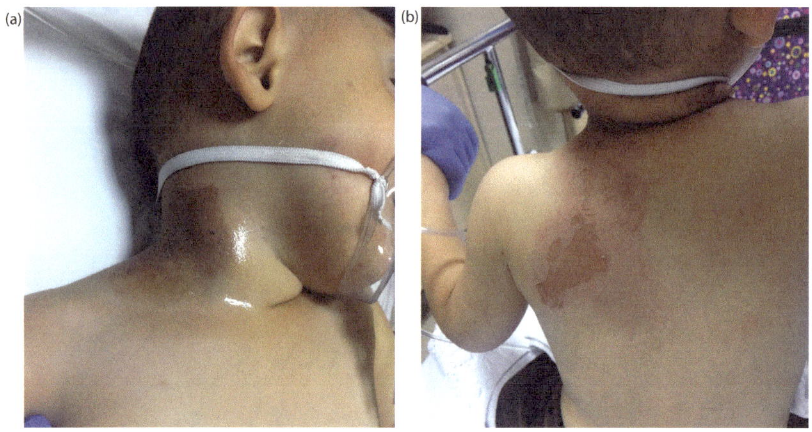

Figure 2. Injury of the neck (a) and back (b) resulting from casting onto the skin during caustic ingestion.

Long-term complications usually develop 3 weeks after the injury. Most commonly, strictures occur due to increased fibrosis in the injured area. The esophagus is the most severely affected gastrointestinal segment in most caustic ingestion patients. Therefore, the majority of upper gastrointestinal strictures secondary to caustic ingestion develop in the esophagus. Esophageal strictures may involve a short segment (usually accepted as shorter than two vertebral bodies in length) or a long segment (described as more than two vertebral bodies in length), or even the whole esophagus [38, 39] (**Figure 3a–d**). The rate of esophageal stricture has been reported to be between 2 and 63% in different series [2, 13, 29, 40–42]. Baskin et al. reported that 4.7% of grade-2a injured patients and 26% of grade 2b injured patients

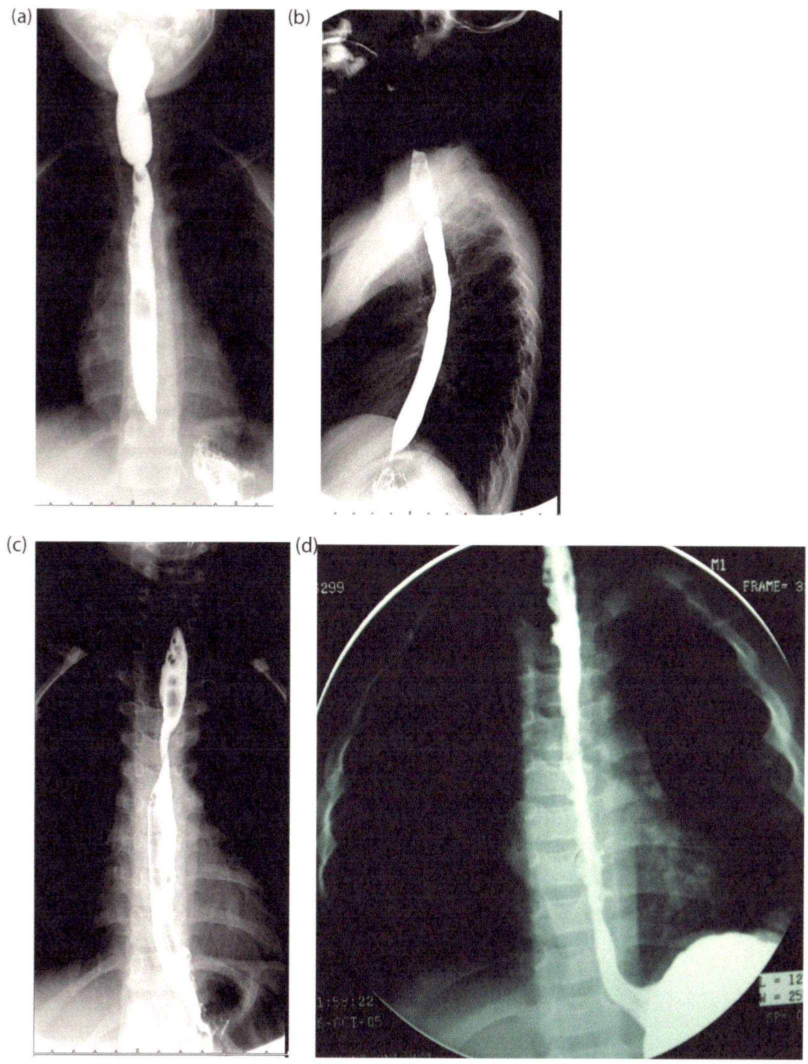

Figure 3. Barium meal studies reveal short segment (a and b) and long segment (c and d) stricture of esophagus in 7 years old boy and 15 years old girl respectively.

develop esophageal strictures [29]. Huang et al. reported that all grade 2 and 3 injured patients develop esophageal strictures [40]. Temiz et al. showed an esophageal stricture rate of 32.1 and 100%, respectively, in patients with grade 2b and 3 injuries [5]. The second most common level of upper gastrointestinal stricture due to caustic ingestion is the pylorus (**Figure 4**). This usually occurs due to accumulation of the ingested substance at the antrum or pylorus level. Several studies have reported that the overall incidence of gastric outlet obstruction is between 5 and 10% [12, 43–45]. Temiz et al. showed a pyloric obstruction rate of 15.7% in patients with severe gastric injury [5]. Gastric outlet obstruction may present with gastroesophageal reflux symptoms. The third long-term complication of caustic ingestion is gastroesophageal reflux and hiatal hernia (**Figure 5**). It occurs as a result of esophageal shortening and retraction due to the inflammation and fibrosis that develop secondary to the ingestion injury. Progressive inflammation and fibrosis may cause disruption of His' angle and even a hiatal hernia. This clinical presentation may cause growth retardation or the inability to eat. Also, gastroesophageal reflux may increase the rate of esophageal stricture and influence the response to the treatment of esophageal stricture.

Esophageal carcinoma is another long-term complication [46–48]. This is usually squamous cell carcinoma. Appelqvist and Salmo showed in patients that had ingested lye (the mean age of patients at the time of lye ingestion was 6.2) that the mean latent period between ingestion and esophageal carcinoma was 41 years [46]. Moreover, 84% of these patients had squamous cell carcinoma at the middle part of esophagus. Kochhar et al. reported two patients with esophageal carcinoma after acidic agent ingestion [49]. Patients with esophageal strictures secondary to caustic ingestion have more than a 1000-fold risk of

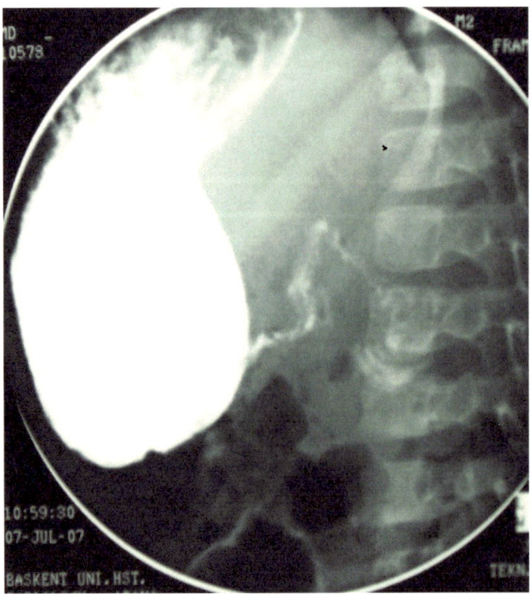

Figure 4. Barium meal study reveals pyloric stenosis secondary to the acidic substance ingestion.

http://dx.doi.org/10.5772/67526

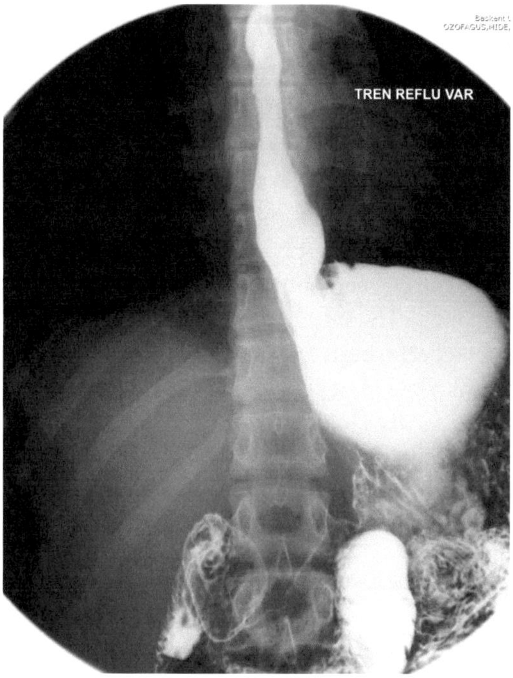

Figure 5. Gastroesophageal reflux and sliding type of hiatal hernia is presented by contrast study.

developing esophageal carcinoma [49]. Appelqvist et al. reviewed a total of 2414 patients with esophageal carcinoma and found that 2.6% of them had a history of caustic injury of the esophagus [46].

4. Diagnostic methods

Several techniques and methods, including laboratory tests, radiological studies, scintigraphy, and endoscopy, are used to determine the severity and depth of injury.

4.1. Laboratory

White blood cell count, C-reactive protein, plasma creatinine level, aspartate aminotransferase (AST), alanine aminotransferase (ALT), and blood gases are usually assessed in serious cases. These tests can be used both in diagnosis and in management to define whether the patient has developed complications. High white blood cell counts (>20,000 cells/mm^3), low arterial pH (<7.22), and low base excess (< −12) are considered signs of serious esophageal injury in adults [50, 51]. However there is no clinical study that examined the relation of laboratory findings and caustic injury level. Laboratory tests are also used for the detection and monitoring of systemic and metabolic complications such as liver damage or renal insufficiency [28].

4.2. Endoscopy

Several studies have indicated that clinical signs are not helpful in predicting the degree of injury and late complications. However, the necessity for endoscopy has been discussed in the literature previously; esophagogastroduodenoscopy is still the most preferred and effective diagnostic practice and approach [4, 5, 28, 53] It is based on direct visualization and staging of injury according to the grading system previously described. It can be performed using a rigid or flexible endoscope. While only the esophagus can be seen by rigid endoscopes, both the esophagus and the stomach can be seen with a flexible endoscope. It is recommended within the first 24–48 hours after injury. The burned area of the esophagus is weakest between days 7 and 21 after injury [2]. Due to the high frequency of complications related with endoscopy, such as fistulas, perforation or bleeding, it is not recommended in patients with high grade injuries [2]. Moreover, it is usually recommended to stop endoscopy at the first severe circumferential burn because of the risk of complications [2, 52]. Poley et al. reported that the esophagus was the most severely affected segment of the upper gastrointestinal tract in 79% of their patients [28]. Injury to the stomach, especially the fundus and body, was relatively common. They observed damage to the duodenum only in 6% of their patients [28]. Doğan et al. observed gastric injury in 17.1% of patients [53]. Urgancı et al. reported normal or mild injury (57%), severe esophagitis (19.1%), erosive gastritis (4.3%), gastric necrosis (0.3%), esophagogastritis (3.7%), and esophagogastroduodenitis (4%) in their series [4]. Temiz et al. reported that 18.4% of patients with severe esophageal injury likewise had severe gastric injury (**Figure 6a–d**). Also, 3.4% of their patients had more severe damage to the stomach than to the esophagus [5]. They performed complete upper gastrointestinal endoscopy to avoid overlooking a gastric injury, even in patients with severe esophageal damage. They reported that there were no complications due to late or complete endoscopy, even in severely damaged patients [5]. There are many articles about esophageal endoscopic findings, but there are limited studies providing gastric findings after caustic ingestion in children [5, 28]. Poley reported that normal findings or mild esophageal injury was found in 40% of patients, while this value was 80% in a study by Boskovic [15, 28]. Doğan et al. reported normal or mild injury in 47.5% of patients [53]. Temiz et al. reported that 43.2% of their patients had normal or mild esophagitis demonstrated by endoscopy, while they all presented with positive clinical findings [5]. In this way, unnecessary hospitalization was prevented by endoscopy [5, 15, 28]. Also, endoscopy can be used for planning the treatment of possible complications such as early dilation of the esophagus in severely injured patients [5, 54]. Radiologically suspected or proven gastrointestinal perforations, severe respiratory injury with distress, poor general condition or metabolic imbalance are accepted as contraindications of endoscopy. However, endoscopy can be performed under sedation within a short period of time. The rate of complications related to endoscopy is very low. Bleeding, perforation, and mucosal tears are complications of endoscopy. Iqbal et al. reported a 0.06% rate of complications in all endoscopy procedures, regardless of the indication [55]. Although Doğan et al. reported that esophageal perforation occurred after endoscopy in one patient (0.21%), most of the articles which examined the results of endoscopy in caustic ingestion patients reported no complications [5, 15, 28, 53]. Although many articles have emphasized the importance of early endoscopy in planning the treatment strategy, some centers do not offer early endoscopic examination, claiming that

http://dx.doi.org/10.5772/67526

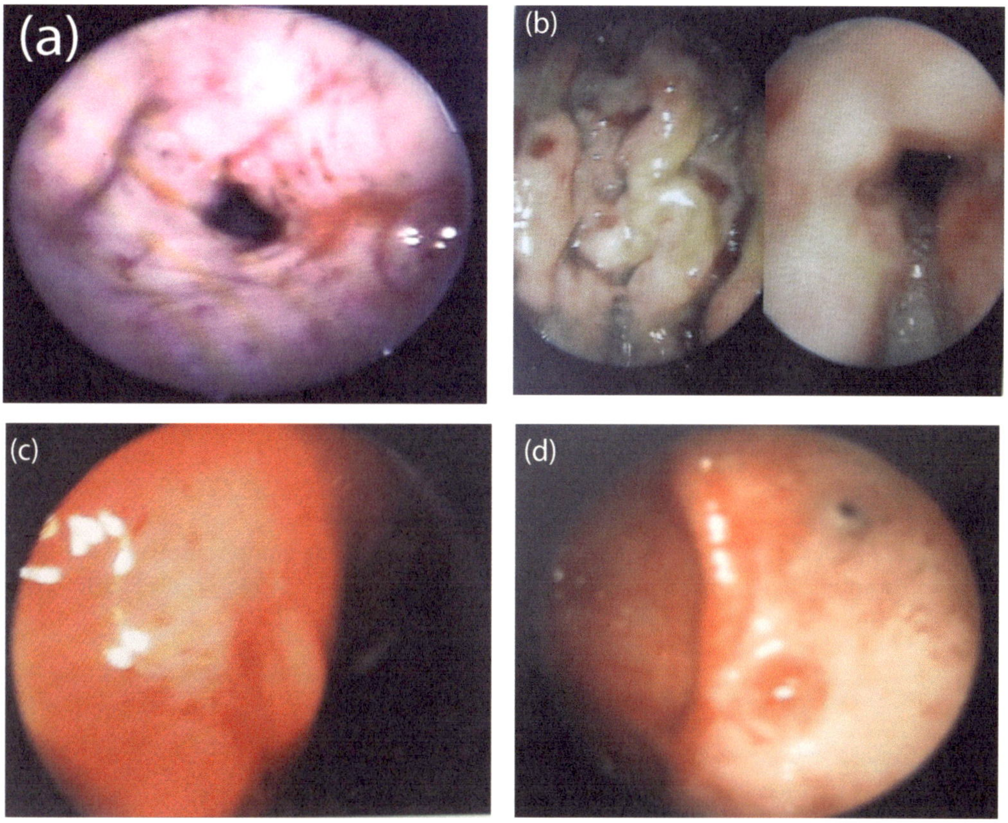

Figure 6. Endoscopy demonstrated the severe caustic injury in the esophagus (a) antrum and pylorus (b). Pylorus narrowing was observed in the control endoscopy (c). A pint point appearance of pylorus in a patient admitted during the past period (d).

endoscopic findings do not change treatment strategies [14, 42, 56]. Additionally, the risk of general anesthesia and the complications of endoscopy are avoided using these protocols [42]. Lamireau et al. reported that the absence of symptoms was always associated with no or minimal lesions in their patients. Therefore, they did not recommend endoscopy in asymptomatic patients, especially in developed countries [14]. In the same way, Gupta et al. reported that all patients with clinically significant injuries were symptomatic. Also, all asymptomatic patients had normal findings on endoscopic examinations [56].

4.3. Scintigraphy

In the last two decades, clinical and experimental studies have been performed assessing the value of scintigraphic evaluation and detection of caustic injury of the esophagus [57, 58]. Millar et al. performed a prospective clinical study to assess whether sucralfate has an affinity for the chemically injured esophagus and to assess the accuracy of radiolabeled sucralfate as an indicator of the presence and extent of esophageal injury [57]. They found that technetium-99m scintigraphy is an accurate diagnostic method to assess caustic esophageal injury [57]. Technetium-99m pyrophosphate scintigraphy has been used in diagnostic studies on the detection of caustic esophageal injury [58, 59].

In the late period, scintigraphic studies may be used to evaluate esophageal transit time, gastric emptying and gastroesophageal reflux, which are common complications [60]. Technetium-99m sulfur colloid in milk or formula is often used for gastrointestinal scintigraphic studies [61]. Kochhar et al. performed a study to assess esophageal motor dysfunction in patients with corrosive esophageal stricture. They used segmental and total esophagus transit time. They found that esophageal transit time is prolonged in one-third of patients with corrosive injury-induced esophageal strictures despite adequate esophageal dilatation. They also reported that these findings were correlated with the length of the stricture and the severity of dysphagia [62].

4.4. Radiology

Several radiological modalities are used to define early and late complications. These studies vary from simple plain chest or abdominal X-ray to complex contrast studies such as cine esophagography or computerized tomography.

4.4.1. Chest X-ray, erect abdominal X-ray

Pneumothorax, pneumomediastinum, or pneumoperitoneum, which are signs of esophageal or gastric perforation, can be observed. These methods are often used in patients with hematemesis.

4.4.2. Esophagogastrography

This is useful for the demonstration of early or late complications. Esophageal stenosis, hiatal hernia, gastroesophageal reflux, pyloric stenosis, esophageal perforation, gastric perforation or tracheoesophageal fistula can be demonstrated with contrast studies. Traditional esophagography may not show pathology in some cases. In these situations, cine esophagography may be helpful (**Figure 7**). In suspected patients, the uses of water-soluble substances, which are less irritant than barium, are preferred for the demonstration of esophageal or gastric perforation (**Figure 8**). However, more radiologic details with better images are obtained with barium meal studies. Contrast studies are also used to determine the location and length of the esophageal stricture (**Figure 9a** and **b**).

4.4.3. Ultrasonography (US)

There have been some studies that focused on the utility of endoscopic esophageal or gastric miniprobe US to predict of outcomes of caustic injury [63–66]. The basis for this method is to evaluate the integrity of the mucosa and deeper muscle layers or to assess gastric wall thickness. Endoscopic ultrasonographic findings are classified as grade-1 when involving only the mucosal edema and grade-2 and grade-3 with destruction of the muscular layers. Grades 2

http://dx.doi.org/10.5772/67526

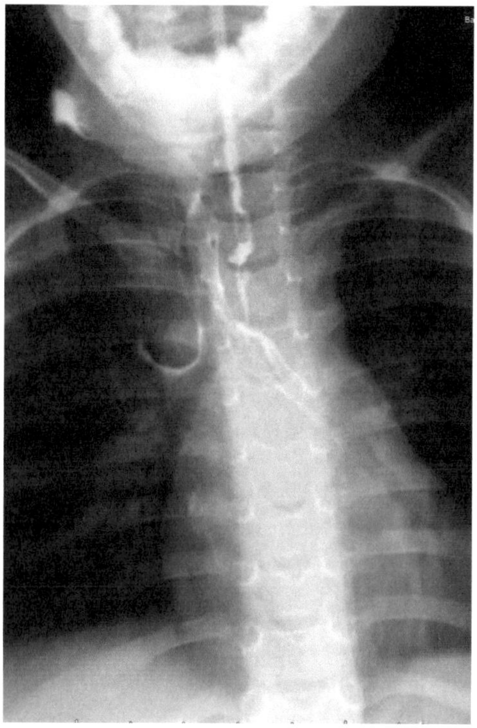

Figure 7. Tracheoesophageal fistula was described by cine esophagography.

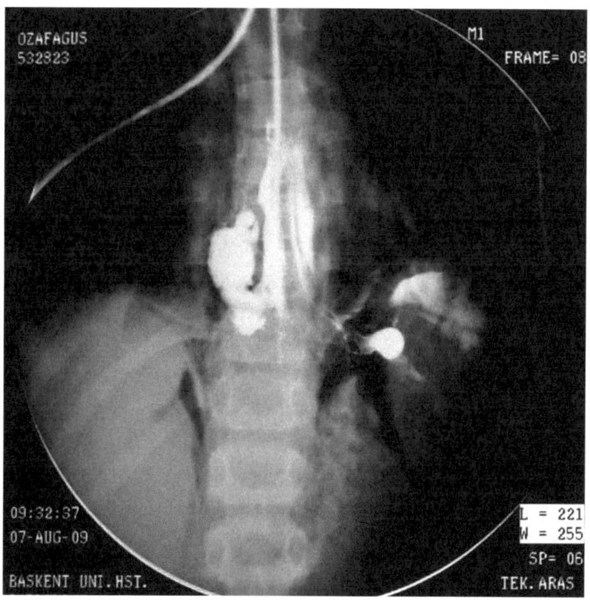

Figure 8. Contrast meal study revealed esophageal perforation after dilatation session.

(a) (b)

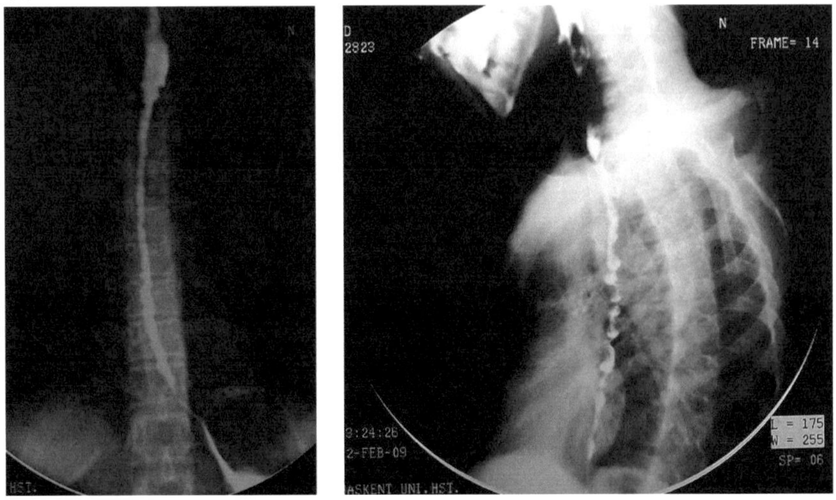

Figure 9. (a) and (b) Multiple and long segment strictures of esophagus were showed by esophagography.

and 3 are associated with the development of future esophageal or gastric strictures [63–66]. However, Chiu et al. reported that US does not increase the accuracy of predicting early or late complications when used in conjunction with conventional endoscopic observation [66].

4.4.4. Computerized tomography (CT)

CT is usually used to define transmural injury and the extent of necrosis in patients with complications such as esophageal or gastric perforations due to caustic ingestion. Ryu et al. recently described a grading system to predict late complications after caustic ingestion [30].

5. Treatment

The treatment approach to caustic ingestion can be divided into two stages: acute management and the treatment of complications.

5.1. Acute management

The acute management of caustic ingestion is based on the general principles of acute trauma life support guidelines. The aim of this approach is the stabilization of vital functions. This includes continuity of the airway and respiratory function and controlling the circulation. Hemodynamic and respiratory stabilization should be priority aims. Endotracheal intubation may be necessary in patients with severe airway caustic injury. Intubation can be difficult in patients with a severely affected airway. Fiber optic laryngoscopy may provide direct

http://dx.doi.org/10.5772/67526

visualization and safe intubation. Thus, the complications that occur secondary to blind intubation may be prevented [6, 10]. Oral feeding is discontinued and adequate intravenous fluid replacement should be provided [10, 31]. A detailed history and identification and measurement of the pH level of the ingested caustic substance will provide information about the severity of the injury. Chest and erect abdominal X-ray should be performed to look for pneumomediastinum, pneumothorax, and pneumoperitoneum, which indicate esophageal or gastric perforation. pH neutralization is not recommended, because it can increase damage by direct effects on the mucosa. This may also cause emesis and vomiting, which may cause recurrent injury to the esophagus [10]. Nasogastric decompression is recommended to prevent vomiting and to provide gastric decompression. However, the benefits have not been conclusively shown. It may be used as a stent in severe circumferential injury. The placement of nasogastric tubes is recommended under endoscopic visualization to prevent esophageal perforation. Oral feeding is still controversial. The authors who believe in the necessity of endoscopy recommend feeding after endoscopy if the findings are normal or mild [5, 53]. In patients with severe esophagitis, enteral nutrition may be applied via a nasogastric tube. However, some authors prefer enteral nutrition without endoscopy for patients who are able to swallow their saliva easily [42]. They perform barium contrast esophagography after 3 weeks. In cases of esophageal or gastric stricture, endoscopy and dilatation are performed [42]. Total parenteral nutrition is preferred in patients with severe gastric injury or who are intolerant to enteral nutrition with normal gastroscopic findings [5, 42]. Proton pump inhibitors or H_2 antagonists are usually recommended to prevent possible gastroesophageal injury or stress ulcers [25, 29, 31]. However, the beneficial effects of agents that reduce gastric pH levels remain unclear. Broad spectrum antibiotics are preferred by many authors, especially in patients with airway injury [5, 6, 25]. However, there is no evidence that antibiotics reduce infections of the injured area or the rate of stricture formation. The benefits of corticosteroids are still controversial. Two different studies that presented a meta-analysis of the literature regarding the use of corticosteroids in caustic injury showed that steroids do not have beneficial effects [67, 68]. Anderson et al. found that there is no benefit from the use of steroids in caustic injured patients regarding the rate of stricture formation [69]. However, there are also studies presenting the opposite opinion. Mamede et al. found that antibiotics combined with corticosteroids reduced the incidence of stenosis [70]. These authors reported infection and gastrointestinal bleeding as side effects of corticosteroids, especially in patients who had ingested large amounts of a caustic substance. Bautista et al. also reported that dexamethasone had better effects than prednisone [71]. Usta et al. investigated the effects of a high dose methylprednisolone (1 g/1.73 m^2) on caustic esophageal burns [72]. They found that the stricture development rate and the duration of total parenteral nutrition were statistically significantly low in the methylprednisolone group [72]. Boukthir et al. reported that high dose methylprednisolone seems to improve the prognosis and prevent stricture formation in grade-2b injured patients [73]. Another situation is the treatment of metabolic complications of caustic injury including renal insufficiency, hepatic dysfunction, diffuse intravascular coagulation, and hemolysis or acute pancreatitis. Supportive care and medication are important [28]. Blood and blood product replacement, hemodialysis and other medications are arranged depending on the clinical and laboratory findings of the patient.

5.2. Treatment of complications

5.2.1. Acute complications

The most severe acute complications are esophageal and gastric perforations. These complications are diagnosed by regular chest or abdominal X-ray. Esophageal perforation is commonly described in adult patients. Aggressive surgical interventions such as esophagectomy or esophagostomy are recommended in adults with esophageal perforation [74, 75]. It is known that more conservative treatment modalities are preferred in several diseases in children. Tube thoracostomy into the pleural space or mediastinum may be performed. However, gastric perforation due to caustic ingestion is more often reported than esophageal perforation in children [76–78]. It is diagnosed by a pneumoperitoneum under the diaphragm and requires immediate surgery. Partial or total gastrectomy with roux-n-y gastrojejunostomy or esophagojejunostomy or different gastrointestinal reconstruction procedures may required.

5.2.2. Esophageal stricture

Esophageal stricture is most serious complication of caustic ingestion. It usually occurs in patients with grade 2a and more severe injury. Various treatment approaches ranging from minimally invasive methods such as balloon dilatation to aggressive surgery such as colonic transposition have been described.

5.2.2.1. Dilatation

Bougienage has traditionally been used as a first step in the treatment of esophageal stricture. Bougienage can be performed both antegradely by using Savary-Gilliard dilatators over a guide wire and retrogradely via gastrostomy. Balloon dilatation has recently become the most common and preferred method of dilatation [38, 79–81]. The dilatation force is applied equally and radially at the esophageal wall with balloon dilatation; rigid dilatators induce axial, radial, and shearing force [80, 82]. Balloon dilation can be performed easily with low complication rates in experienced hands. Esophageal perforation is the most serious complication of esophageal balloon dilatation and has been reported to occur in 0.33–45% of balloon dilatation sessions in previous studies [38, 80, 83, 84]. Esophageal perforations usually occur in patients with delayed treatment or with long segment strictures that have become fibrotic. Esophageal perforations that occur secondary to dilatation are almost always treated with a conservative approach [38, 76, 79]. Respiratory distress, fever, or severe chest pain could cause a perforation after dilatation. Chest X-ray may reveal pneumothorax or pneumomediastinum. Treatment with broad spectrum antibiotics and the interruption of feeding are the initial treatment steps. Chest tube insertion may be required in respiratory distress or in the presence of pleural effusion. However, complication rates can be reduced by using a staged dilatation, i.e., gradually increasing the diameter over consecutive sessions to the required balloon diameter with experienced hands [38, 79]. It is known as remodeling time; stabilization of the esophageal stricture requires between 6 months and 3 years. In light of this information, long-term dilatation may be required in severe cases [38, 85]. Gündoğdu et al. reported that the success rate of conservative approach was higher in patients younger than 8 years of age, and in strictures due to caustics other than lye involving upper third portion and less than 5 cm of length [85]. Repeated hospitalization and general anesthesia are accepted as disadvantages of long-term dilatation. Doo et al. reported a 91% technical success rate and a 64% clinical success rate [84]. Kim et al. obtained a 100% technical success rate and a 46% clinical success rate in their patients [39]. However, Alshammari et al. reported a 33% failure rates for balloon dilatation of caustic esophageal strictures [86]. Temiz et al. reported the results of long-term dilatation up to 4 years; full recovery occurred with long-term dilatation [38]. The author suggested that balloon dilatation is a safe and effective method and that the dilatation program should be carried out for at least 2 years before deciding that dilatation has failed [38]. Tiryaki et al. reported their experience with early prophylactic bougienage methods. They found that the strictures had resolved after 6 months of dilatation in patients initially treated prophylactically with early bougienage, whereas stricture resolution did not occur for more than 1 year in patients in whom dilatation began after stricture development [54]. Uygun et al. evaluated their early and late dilatation results in patients with short and long segments caustic esophageal strictures [79]. They reported a 100% success rate. Also, they reported that treatment with early balloon dilatation was significantly faster and shorter than that in the late dilatation group, and short stricture treatment was also of significantly shorter duration than long stricture treatment [79]. However, there are no controlled data to support the use of early dilatation, which could increase the risk of perforation [87].

Balloon dilatation is usually performed as one dilatation every 3 weeks for the first 3 months with subsequent modifications as required thereafter [88]. However, the patient's complaints and clinical condition are the most influential factor on the frequency of sessions. Temiz et al. reported that dilatations were performed weekly initially [38]. Eventually, balloon dilatation will be accepted as a safe and effective treatment modality with a low rate of complications for caustic esophageal strictures [38, 42, 79, 89].

5.2.2.1.1. Balloon dilatation technique

This operation is performed under general anesthesia. The radiopaque guide wire is introduced fluoroscopically or endoscopically to the stomach. The balloon catheter is pushed over the wire and placed in the stricture. Then, the balloon is inflated with radiocontrast solution. The balloon is inflated until a flattening of the hourglass deformity of the stricture observed for 2–4 minutes [38, 42] (**Figure 10a–c**). The same procedure is applied at each location for multiple or long segment strictures. The first dilatation starts with the smallest balloon even 4 or 6 mm diameter. The balloon sizes are increased to the appropriate diameter equal to the patient's esophageal diameter, defined by the thumb rule, i.e., the esophageal diameter is equal to the diameter of the patient's own thumb [42, 90].

5.2.2.2. Stenting

Intraluminal esophageal stenting is an option in cases of intractable strictures. It should be mentioned that stenting should be continued until complete esophageal healing. Therefore, stenting is a long-term treatment strategy. Mutaf reported outcomes with polytetrafluorethylene stents

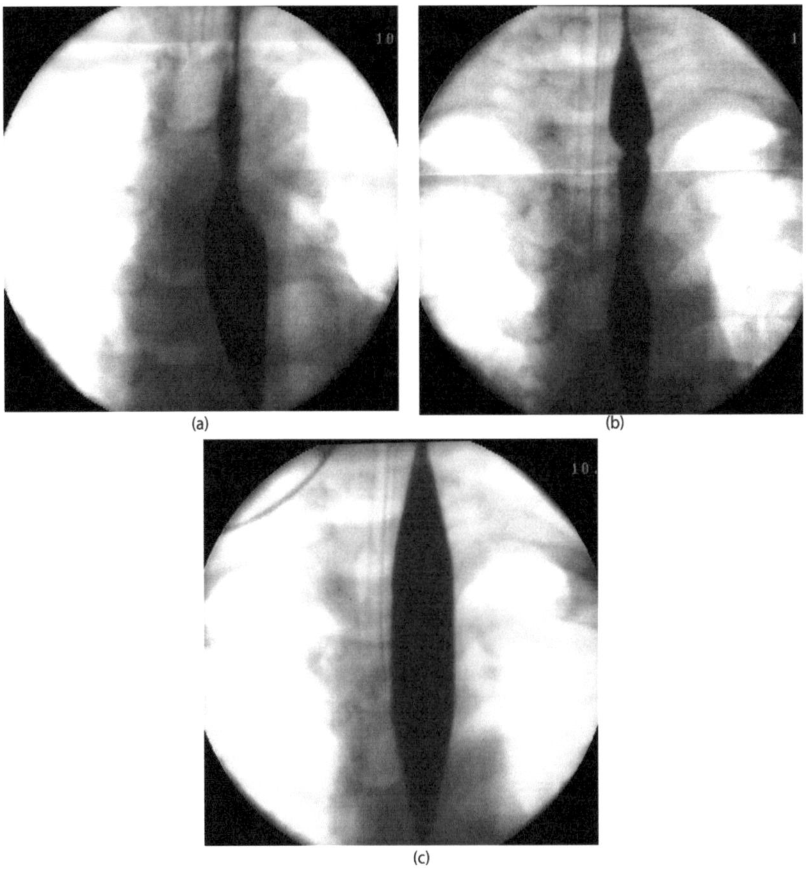

Figure 10. (a)–(c) The balloon catheter is pushed over the wire and placed in the stricture. Then, the balloon is inflated with radiocontrast solution until a flattening of the hourglass deformity.

5 mm in diameter or larger [88]. The stent was replaced with a 1 mm larger stent every third week, and was left in place for 1 year after a stent diameter of 10 mm was reached. However, stent placement is usually applied after dilatation session in different series [91–93]. Using this method, a success rate of 68% was reported. Atabek et al. also reported that 72.7% of their patients resumed normal feeding after 9–14 months of stenting. So, long-term stenting is an effective method to reduce the necessity for major surgical intervention for recalcitrant esophageal strictures [91]. Foschia et al. reported an 86.6% success rate with dynamic stents. They claimed that stenting reduces the necessity of dilatation sessions [92]. Gastroesophageal reflux and poor patient compliance are the most commonly encountered causes of stenting failure [88]. However, stents can worsen esophagitis by increasing reflux. The migration of stents, sialorrhea, retching, esophageal subclavian fistula, stent dislocation and perforation, soft plate injury, swallowing difficulties, chest pain, and vomiting are the reported complications [88, 91, 93]. Zhang et al. reported complete improvement in all their limited number of patients with self-expanding stents without serious complications [94]. Recently, self-expandable, biodegradable stents have become available and usable for the treatment of esophageal strictures. Stent integ-

http://dx.doi.org/10.5772/67526

rity and a radial force that continues for 6–8 weeks are seen as the advantages of the approach [87]. However, there have been no controlled trials yet on these stents.

5.2.2.3. *Topical mitomycin C and steroid treatment*

These options are based on their antifibroblastic properties, with a preventive effect on collagen synthesis and chronic scarring [42, 95–97]. El-Asmar et al. performed a double-blinded, randomized, placebo-controlled trial on the effects of topical mitomycin C application in patients with caustic esophageal strictures [98]. They found that topical mitomycin C application statistically significantly reduced the number of dilatation sessions. Mitomycin C is usually recommended at a dose of 0.4 mg/ml, which is applied with cotton or a pledget via a rigid endoscope [98, 99]. Additionally, submucosal application of triamcinolone acetonide, a member of the steroid family, has been used in patients with refractory caustic strictures. It can be applied together with endoscopic dilation [42, 97]. In the treatment approach, 2 ml (40 mg/ml) of triamcinolone acetonide is injected into quadrant 3 or 4 of the esophageal stricture at intervals of 2 or 3 weeks until full recovery [42].

5.2.2.4. *Surgery*

It is well established that the child's own esophagus is the ideal option and the esophagus should be preserved without any replacement for native esophagus [100–103]. The ideal organ to be used for replacement is expected to deliver food efficiently from the mouth to the intestinal system, to be resistant to stomach acid, grow parallel to the child, preserving cardiac and respiratory functions [101, 102]. The indication of esophageal replacement in patients with caustic stricture is failure of normal swallowing [100] (**Figure 11a** and **b**). Although multiple strictures, longer than 5-cm stricture and tortuous strictures, which do not allow to passage of the guidewire are the contraindications of esophageal dilatation, it is still controversial

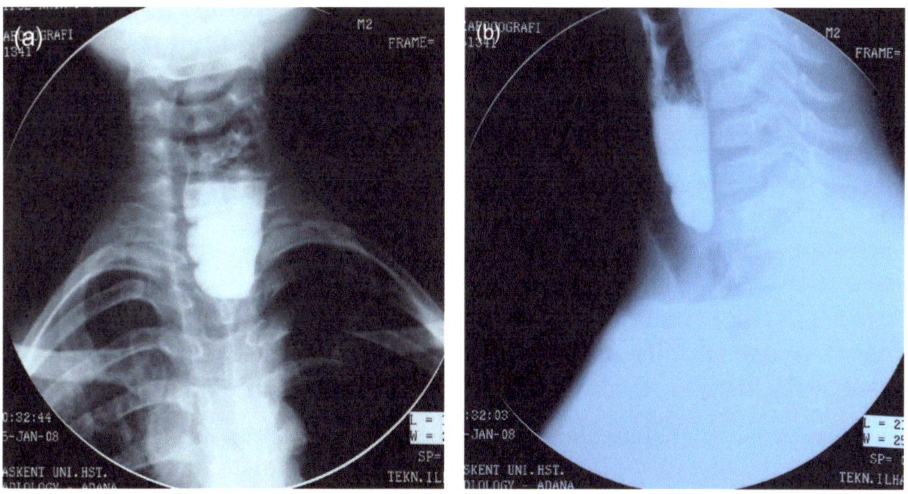

Figure 11. Complete obstruction of the cervical esophagus prevents oral feeding. Posterior-anterior (a) and lateral (b) frame of obstruction.

[38, 100]. Psychological problems may also occur secondary to prolonged dilatation, which required repeated anesthesia are other indications for esophageal replacement [100]. Spitz reported that necessity of regular dilatation for 6–12 months following the ingestion constituted an indication for esophageal replacement in caustic esophageal injury [104]. Gundoğdu et al. suggested that difficulty to swallow saliva, total or nearly total obliteration of the lumen involving more than 3 cm of an esophagus at admittance, difficulty in swallowing within one-month period following the recent dilation after completion of one-year dilation program were the main indications of esophageal replacement [105]. Social and psychological problems due to the lack of normal feeding or swallow, interrupted schooling and domestic family problems secondary to prolonged and multiple hospital admissions may be also considered other reasons of esophageal substations [102].

Surgical techniques include resection and end-to-end anastomosis, colonic or jejunal interposition, reversed gastric tube, or gastric transposition have been described for esophageal replacement in patients with resistant strictures [100, 104, 106]. Although the colon is the most commonly used intestinal component, progressively increased gastric transposition has been reported in recent years. Colonic interposition can be performed in the posterior mediastinum with transhiatal esophagectomy. It can be also done retrosternally by leaving the native esophagus.

Various segments of the colon can be used depending on the discretion of the surgeon [107, 108]. Ergün et al. used the left colon in 75% of their patients, while Bothereau et al. performed right colonic interposition in 87% of their patients [107, 108]. However, the latter authors reported no statistically significant difference in the complication rates [108]. Complications of colonic transposition are also frequently seen. Hamza et al. reported 1% mortality due to postoperative respiratory problems or sepsis [100]. Bothereau et al. reported 4% mortality secondary to complications [108]. Complications are classified under three main titles as early, late, and long-term complications. Early complications are defined as those occurred within the first month of surgery, while late complications are those occurred between 1 month and 1 year after surgery. Complications are described as long-term, while occurring more than 1 year after operation [109]. Complications of colonic interposition are summarized in **Table 2** [100, 107–112]. Cervical anastomotic leakage, adhesive intestinal obstructions, coloesophageal stricture, redundancy, gastrocolic reflux, and graft necrosis are the most common complications (**Figures 12** and **13a** and **b**). Furthermore, several suggestions have been made to reduce the rate of complications. Ergün et al. reported that the incidence of cervical anastomotic stricture was significantly lower by two-stage procedure. Bothereau et al. showed the upper thoracic inlet enlargement by resection of manubrium and tip of left clavicle to reduce the rate of complications in colonic interposition [108]. Also, Chirica et al. reported that the absence of thoracic inlet enlargement, delayed reconstruction were associated with an increased risk of early and late complications in adults [113].

Gastric transposition is another choice of surgical treatment. The method popularized by Spitz et al. which is the largest-scale study, has been increasingly utilized in recent years [103]. It is based on the good blood supply of the stomach. The right gastric and gastroepiploic vessels are preserved, and the left gastric and left gastroepiploic vessels are ligated. After the stomach is fully mobilized and passed transhiatal, posterior mediastinally, fundus

http://dx.doi.org/10.5772/67526

Intraoperative complication	Pneumothorax
	Tracheal injury
	Major bleeding
	Recurrent laryngeal injury
Early complications	Death
	Greft necrosis
	Respiratory failure
	Gstrocolic reflux
	Sepsis
	Fistula
	Cervical anastomotic stricture
	Cologastric anastomosis stricture
	Dehiscence of colocolic anastomosis
	Dehiscence of cologastric anastomosis
	Dumping syndrome
	Intussusception
	Enterocutaneous fistula
	Biliary reflux
Late complications	Anastomotic stricture
	Reflux
	Redundancy
	Ulceration
	Greft hernia into the pleura
	Intestinal obstruction
	Aspiration pneumonia
	Incisional hernia
	Postprandial neck bulge
Long-term complication	Relux
	Dysphagia
	Pain
	Nocturnal regurgitation
	Redundancy
	Anastomotic stricture
	Ulceration
	Scoliosis
	Malnutrition

Table 2. Complications of colonic interposition [100, 107–112].

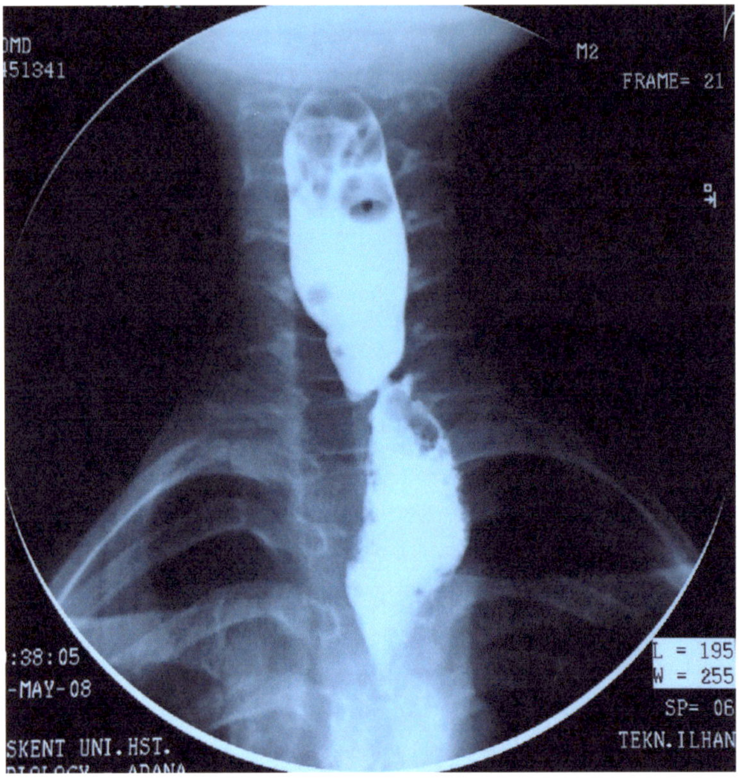

Figure 12. Coloesophageal stricture in a 14 years old girl underwent colonic interposition.

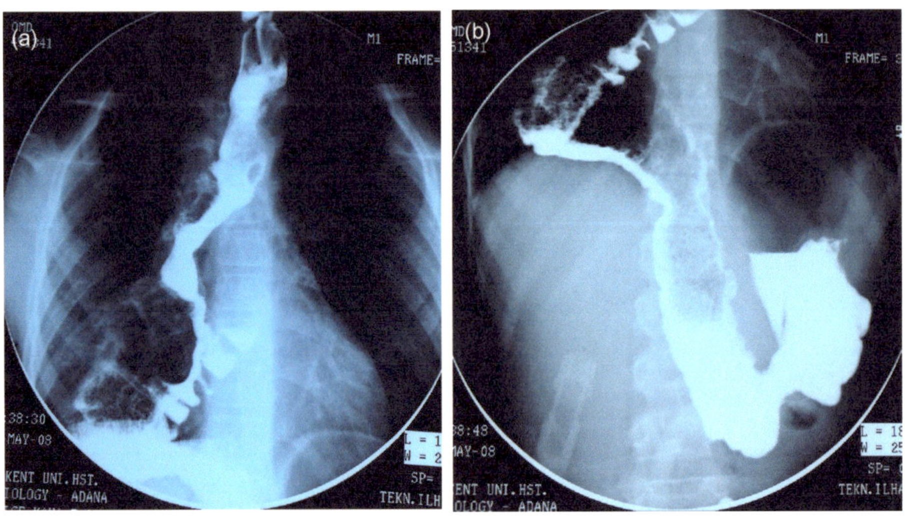

Figure 13. Colonic redundancy after coloesophagoplasty. Thoracic (a) and abdominal (b) appearance.

is pulled up from the cervical incision. Anastomosis between the stomach and esophagus is performed between the gastric fundus, which is easily mobilized and has a good blood supply and the cervical esophagus. Pyloroplasty or pyloromyotomy is carried out with the aim of facilitating gastric emptying [101, 102, 104]. Gastric transposition can usually be performed without thoracotomy. Spitz et al. performed thoracotomy in selected patients, due to dense fibrous tissues [114]. The most common complications of total gastric transposition up are the anastomotic leakage, stenosis, swallowing disorders, delayed gastric emptying, and mortality [101, 103, 114, 115]. Anastomotic leakage usually resolves spontaneously, while it requires surgical correction in a few cases [114, 115]. Stenosis usually improves with a number of dilatation sessions [114, 115]. Spitz reported that 94% of patients with swallowing difficulties experienced major swallowing problems before the gastric transposition. Severe gastric emptying problem may require converting to the pyloroplasty or Roux-en-Y gastrojejunostomy [103]. Spitz found the result of gastric transpositions to be good to excellent in terms of absence of swallowing difficulties or other gastrointestinal symptoms in 90% of their patients [114]. In another study, Marujo reported excellent and good results in 85 and 15% of patients, respectively [115]. In addition, Angotti et al. reported that all patients had gain weight and height postoperatively [101]. Davenport et al. also reported the long-term results of gastric transposition and showed that gastric transposition allowed satisfactory growth and nutrition for the majority of children [116]. The authors also observed respiratory symptoms in a number of patients and suggested that respiratory symptoms were related to small lung volume, rather than an increased airway resistance. In another study, Tannuri et al. compared esophagocoloplasty and gastric transposition in terms of early complications and mortality [117]. The authors reported that minor complications were statistically significantly higher in colonic transposition, while the rate of major complications was statistically significantly higher in gastric transposition. However, they found no significant difference in the mortality rates between the groups. Hence, they recommended esophagocoloplasty based on their experiences.

5.2.3. Gastric outlet obstruction

Gastric injury is less encountered than esophageal injury in caustic ingestion. Gastric outlet obstruction may develop as early as 3 weeks or as late as 10 weeks [118]. Endoscopy is recommended to diagnose the gastric injury and to tailor the treatment modality. There are two different approaches including minimal invasive technique, endoscopic balloon dilatation of the obstruction, and surgical intervention to resolve the obstructions [43, 45, 119, 120].

5.2.3.1. Endoscopic dilatation

On the other hand, there is limited experience on endoscopic treatment of gastric outlet obstruction secondary to the caustic ingestion in children. Treem et al. reported successful treatment outcomes of pyloric obstruction secondary to caustic ingestion with endoscopy-guided balloon dilatation before three decades. Nasr et al. also reported two patients who underwent endoscopic dilatation; one of them improved only with dilatation. Dehghani et al. reported a patient with pyloric stenosis treated with balloon dilatation [118]. The authors achieved normal pyloric canal after four dilatation sessions. In another study, Temiz et al. attempted endoscopic dilatation in seven patients with corrosive stricture, and performed successful dilatation in five of them [119]. However, symptoms of pyloric obstruction recurred in three patients. Due to the inability to pass the guidewire through the pylorus, they were unable to reperform dilatation. Despite low successful rates, the authors recommended endoscopic balloon dilatation before a surgical intervention.

5.2.3.2. Technique of balloon dilatation

Endoscopy is performed under general anesthesia. After focusing on the pylorus, a radiopaque guidewire is inserted through the pylorus under the guidance of endoscopy. A balloon catheter is passed over the guidewire and through the pylorus. The location of the balloon is monitored endoscopically. Then, the balloon is inflated with a radiopaque solution under fluoroscopic guidance. Inflation is performed for at least 2 minutes after the expansion of hourglass deformity of the obstruction [119] (**Figure 14a–c**).

5.2.3.3. Surgical options

To date, several surgical techniques including Heicke-Mikulicz pyloroplasty, Finney pyloroplasty, Jabulay pyloroplasty, gastrojejunostomy, and Billroth-I procedure have been described for the treatment of acquired gastric outlet obstructions [12, 119, 120]. The preference may vary depending on the discretion of the surgeon. Ozcan et al. performed retrocolic gastrojejunostomy in all patients, while Ozokutan et al. performed gastroduodenostomy and Billroth-I procedure [45, 120]. However, the timing of surgery is of utmost importance for the method to be selected. Surgical intervention is recommended at the end of cicatrization period of caustic injury [44, 119, 121]. Due to anastomotic stricture, secondary to the progressive inflammatory process may develop in early operated patients. Temiz et al. reported anastomotic stricture in a case that underwent gastrojejunostomy after 6 weeks of injury. Endoscopic dilatation may help to solve this problem [119] (**Figure 15a** and **b**). Dumping syndrome is another postoperative clinical condition. Ozcan suggested an anastomosis not exceeding 2 cm to prevent postoperative dumping syndrome [45].

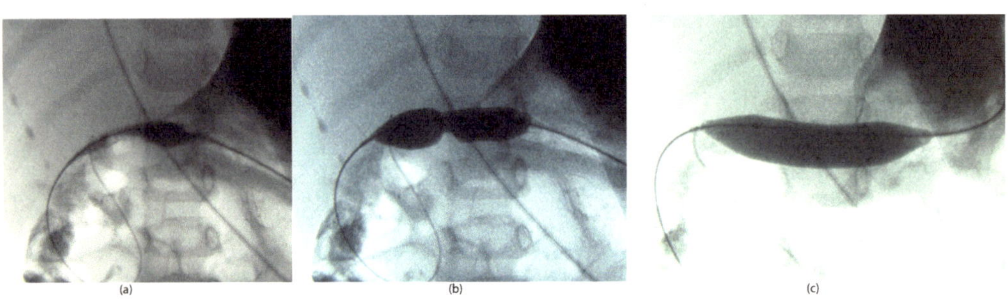

Figure 14. (a)–(c) After placement of guide wire under endoscopic guidance through the pyloric stenosis, a balloon catheter is passed over the guidewire and inflated with radiocontrast solution until a flattening of the hourglass deformity.

http://dx.doi.org/10.5772/67526

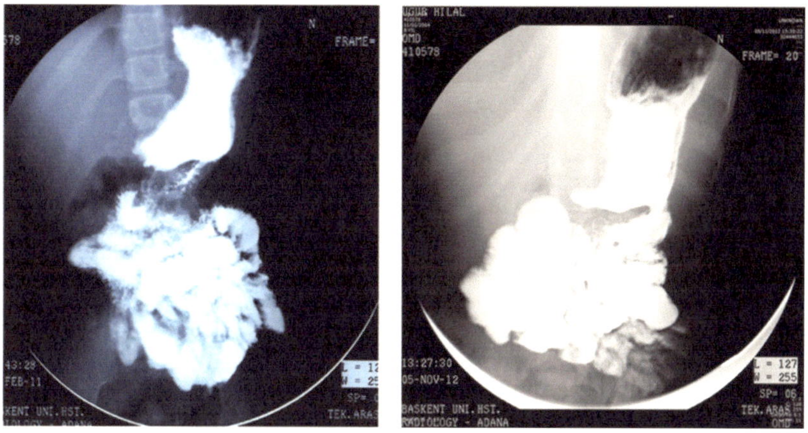

Figure 15. Anastomotic stricture was revealed by gstrography (a), after ballon dilatation easy flow from gastrojejunostomy is seen (b).

5.2.4. Gastroesophageal reflux

Caustic esophageal injury results with narrowed and also shortened esophagus [122]. This process alters the lower esophageal sphincter function, which leads to gastroesophageal reflux. As a consequence, reflux can adversely affect the development of stenosis and response to treatment of the stenosis. Mutaf et al. recommended that patients with caustic esophageal burn should be screened for gastroesophageal reflux during the treatment period [122]. The most preferred surgical procedures for gastroesophageal reflux disease include the Nissen, Thal, and BoixOchoa procedures. However, all these procedures have a significant recurrence rate in the patients, particularly with a shortened esophagus. In addition, Collis gastroplasty with partial or complete fundoplication can be used as alternative surgical techniques in the treatment of a shortened esophagus (**Figure 16a** and **b**).

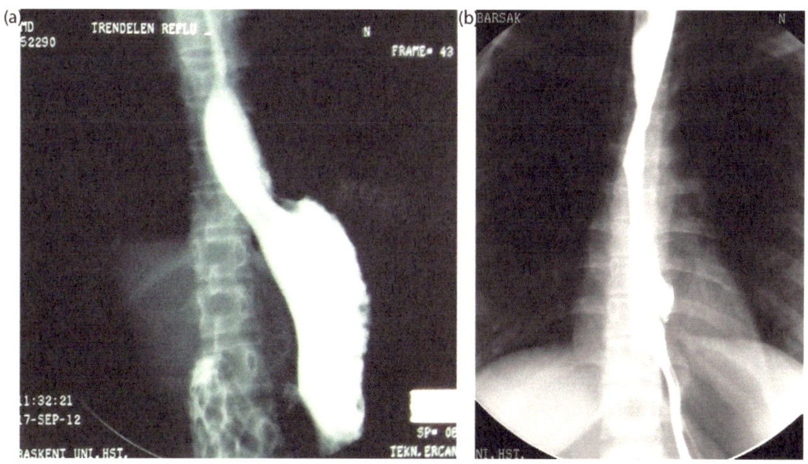

Figure 16. The sliding type of hiatal hernia (a) was ameliorated with Collis gatsroplasty (b).

Author details

Abdulkerim Temiz

Address all correspondence to: aktemiz@yahoo.com

Başkent University, Faculty of Medicine, Department of Pediatric Surgery, Turkey

References

[1] Johnson CM, Brigger MT: The public health impact of pediatric caustic ingestion injuries. Arch Otolaryngol Head Neck Surg. 2012;138:1111–5. doi: 10.1001/jamaoto.2013.672.

[2] de Jong AL, Macdonald R, Ein S, Forte V, Turner A: Corrosive esophagitis in children: a 30-year review. Int J Pediatr Otorhinolaryngol. 2001;57:203–11.

[3] Arévalo-Silva C, Eliashar R, Wohlgelernter J, Elidan J, Gross M: Ingestion of caustic substances: a 15-year experience. Laryngoscope. 2006;116:1422–6.

[4] Urgancı N, Usta M, Kalyoncu D, Demirel E: Corrosive substance ingestion in children. Indian J Pediatr. 2014;81:675–9. doi: 10.1007/s12098-013-1170-0.

[5] Temiz A, Oguzkurt P, Ezer SS, Ince E, Hicsonmez A: Predictability of outcome of caustic ingestion by esophagogastroduodenoscopy in children. World J Gastroenterol. 2012;18:1098–103. doi: 10.3748/wjg.v18.i10.1098.

[6] Lupa M, Magne J, Guarisco JL, Amedee R: Update on the diagnosis and treatment of caustic ingestion. Ochsner J. 2009;9:54–9.

[7] Somuncu S, Cakmak M, Erdogan S, Caglayan O, Akman H, Kaya M: Trapidil, an inhibitor for phosphodiesterase and platelet-derived-growth factor, ameliorates corrosive esophageal burn in rats. Tohoku J Exp Med. 2005;207:203–8.

[8] Ozel SK, Dagli TE, Yuksel M, Kiyan G, Kotiloglu E: The roles of free oxygen radicals, nitric oxide, and endothelin in caustic injury of rat esophagus. J Pediatr Surg. 2004;39:1381–5.

[9] Temiz A, Ünal B, Koçer NE, Oğuzkurt P, Ezer SS, İnce E, Yalçın HS, Hiçsönmez A: Late complications of corrosive esophagitis may be predicted using biochemical methods: preliminary report. Türkiye Klinikleri J Med Sci. 2012;32:193–200. doi:10.5336/medsci.2011-25229.

[10] Contini S, Scarpignato C: Caustic injury of the upper gastrointestinal tract: a comprehensive review. World J Gastroenterol. 2013;19:3918–30. doi:10.3748/wjg.v19.i25.3918.

[11] Mattos GM, Lopes DD, Mamede RC, Ricz H, Mello-Filho FV, Neto JB: Effects of time of contact and concentration of caustic agent on generation of injuries. Laryngoscope. 2006;116:456–60.

[12] Ciftci AO, Senocak ME, Büyükpamukçu N, Hiçsönmez A: Gastric outlet obstruction due to corrosive ingestion: incidence and outcome. Pediatr Surg Int. 1999;15:88–91.

[13] Gaudreault P, Parent M, McGuigan MA, Chicoine L, Lovejoy FH: Predictability of esophageal injury from signs and symptoms: a study of caustic ingestion in 378 children. Pediatrics. 1983;71: 767–70.

[14] Lamireau T, Rebouissoux L, Denis D, Lancelin F, Vergnes P, Fayon M: Accidental caustic ingestion in children: is endoscopy always mandatory? J Pediatr Gastroenterol Nutr. 2001;33:81–4.

[15] Boskovic A, Stankovic I: Predictability of gastroesophageal caustic injury from clinical findings: is endoscopy mandatory in children? Eur J Gastroenterol Hepatol. 2014;26:499–503. doi: 10.1097/MEG.0000000000000060.

[16] Nijhawan S, Jain P: Acute pancreatitis as an unusual complication of corrosive ingestion. J Gastrointestin Liver Dis. 2007;16:345–6.

[17] Gupta V, Kurdia KC, Sharma A, Mishra AK, Yadav TD, Kochhar R: Tracheoesophageal fistula in adults due to corrosive ingestion: challenges in management. Updates Surg. 2015;67:75–81. doi: 10.1007/s13304-015-0292-5.

[18] Samad L, Ali M, Ramzi H: Button battery ingestion: hazards of esophageal impaction. J Pediatr Surg. 1999;34:1527–31.

[19] Marom T, Goldfarb A, Russo E, Roth Y: Battery ingestion in children. Int J Pediatr Otorhinolaryngol. 2010;74:849–54. doi: 10.1016/j.ijporl.2010.05.019.

[20] Votteler TP, Nash JC, Rutledge JC: The hazard of ingested alkaline disk batteries in children. JAMA. 1983;249:2504–6.

[21] Litovitz T, Schmitz BF: Ingestion of cylindrical and button batteries: an analysis of 2382 cases. Pediatrics. 1992;89:747–57.

[22] Bass DH, Millar AJ: Mercury absorption following button battery ingestion. J Pediatr Surg. 1992;27:1541–2.

[23] Hamilton JM, Schraff SA, Notrica DM: Severe injuries from coin cell battery ingestions: 2 case reports. J Pediatr Surg. 2009;44:644–7. doi: 10.1016/j.jpedsurg.2008.10.110.

[24] Loots DP, du Toit-Prinsloo L, Saayman G: Disk battery ingestion: a rare cause of perforation of the brachiocephalic artery. Forensic Sci Med Pathol. 2015;11:614–7. doi: 10.1007/s12024-015-9706-4.

[25] Stiff G, Alwafi A, Rees BI, Lari J: Corrosive injuries of the oesophagus and stomach: experience in management at a regional paediatric centre. Ann R Coll Surg Engl. 1996;78:119–23.

[26] Di Costanzo J, Noirclerc M, Jouglard J, Escoffier JM, Cano N, Martin J, Gauthier A: New therapeutic approach to corrosive burns of the upper gastrointestinal tract. Gut. 1980;21:370–75.

[27] Zargar SA, Kochhar R, Mehta S, Mehta SK: The role of fiberoptic endoscopy in the management of corrosive ingestion and modified endoscopic classification of burns. Gastrointest Endosc. 1991;37:165–9.

[28] Poley JW, Steyerberg EW, Kuipers EJ, Dees J, Hartmans R, Tilanus HW, Siersema PD: Ingestion of acid and alkaline agents: outcome and prognostic value of early upper endoscopy. Gastrointest Endosc. 2004;60:372–7.

[29] Baskin D, Urganci N, Abbasoğlu L, Alkim C, Yalçin M, Karadağ C, Sever N: A standardised protocol for the acute management of corrosive ingestion in children. Pediatr Surg Int. 2004;20:824–8.

[30] Ryu HH, Jeung KW, Lee BK, Uhm JH, Park YH, Shin MH, Kim HL, Heo T, Min YI: Caustic injury: can CT grading system enable prediction of esophageal stricture? Clin Toxicol (Phila). 2010;48:137–42. doi: 10.3109/15563650903585929.

[31] Keh SM, Onyekwelu N, McManus K, McGuigan J: Corrosive injury to upper gastrointestinal tract: still a major surgical dilemma. World J Gastroenterol. 2006;12:5223–8.

[32] Kua K, Jonas N, O'Donnell R: The larynx and caustic soda ingestion. Arch Dis Child. 2015;100:570. doi: 10.1136/archdischild-2014-307588.

[33] Shabino CL, Feinberg A: Esophageal perforation secondary to alkaline battery ingestion. JACEP. 1979;8:360–3.

[34] Chiang MC, Chen YS: Tracheoesophageal fistula secondary to disc battery ingestion. Am J Otolaryngol. 2000;21:333–6.

[35] Anand TS, Kumar S, Wadhwa V, Dhawan R: Rare case of spontaneous closure of tracheo-esophageal fistula secondary to disc battery ingestion. Int J Pediatr Otorhinolaryngol. 2002;63:57–9.

[36] Grisel JJ, Richter GT, Casper KA, Thompson DM: Acquired tracheoesophageal fistula following disc-battery ingestion: can we watch and wait? Int J Pediatr Otorhinolaryngol. 2008;72:699–706. doi: 10.1016/j.ijporl.2008.01.015.

[37] Okuyama H, Kubota A, Oue T, Kuroda S, Nara K, Takahashi T: Primary repair of tracheoesophageal fistula secondary to disc battery ingestion: a case report. J Pediatr Surg. 2004;39:243–4.

[38] Temiz A, Oguzkurt P, Ezer SS, Ince E, Hicsonmez A: Long-term management of corrosive esophageal stricture with balloon dilation in children. Surg Endosc. 2010;24:2287–92. doi: 10.1007/s00464-010-0953-x.

[39] Kim JH, Song HY, Kim HC, Shin JH, Kim KR, Park SW, Jung HY, Lee GH, Park SI: Corrosive esophageal strictures: Long-term effectiveness of balloon dilation in 117 patients. J Vasc Interv Radiol. 2008;19:736–41.

[40] Huang YC, Ni YH, Lai HS, Chang MH: Corrosive esophagitis in children: Pediatr Surg Int. 2004;20:207–10.

[41] Broto J, Asensio M, Jorro CS, Marhuenda C, Vernet JM, Acosta D, Ochoa JB: Conservative treatment of caustic esophageal injuries in children: 20 years of experience. Pediatr Surg Int. 1999;15:323–5.

[42] Bicakci U, Tander B, Deveci G, Rizalar R, Ariturk E, Bernay F: Minimally invasive management of children with caustic ingestion: less pain for patients. Pediatr Surg Int. 2010;26:251–5. doi: 10.1007/s00383-009-2525-5.

[43] Tekant G, Eroğlu E, Erdoğan E, Yeşildağ E, Emir H, Büyükünal C, Yeker D: Corrosive injury-induced gastric outlet obstruction: a changing spectrum of agents and treatment. J Pediatr Surg. 2001;36:1004–7.

[44] Kaushik R, Singh R, Sharma R, Attri AK, Bawa AS: Corrosive-induced gastric outlet obstruction. Yonsei Med J. 2003;44:991–4.

[45] Ozcan C, Ergün O, Sen T, Mutaf O: Gastric outlet obstruction secondary to acid ingestion in children. J Pediatr Surg. 2004;39:1651–3.

[46] Appelqvist P, Salmo M: Lye corrosion carcinoma of the esophagus: a review of 63 cases. Cancer. 1980;45:2655–8.

[47] Kozarek RA, Sanowski RA: Caustic cicatrization of the pharynx associated with dysphagia and premalignant mucosal changes. Am J Gastroenterol. 1982;77:5–8.

[48] Zhang X, Wang M, Han H, Xu Y, Shi Z, Ma G: Corrosive induced carcinoma of esophagus after 58 years. Ann Thorac Surg. 2012;94:2103–5. doi: 10.1016/j.athoracsur.2012.03.110.

[49] Kochhar R, Sethy PK, Kochhar S, Nagi B, Gupta NM: Corrosive induced carcinoma of esophagus: report of three patients and review of literature. J Gastroenterol Hepatol. 2006;21:777–80. doi: 10.1111/j.1440-1746.2006.03211.x.

[50] Rigo GP, Camellini L, Azzolini F, Guazzetti S, Bedogni G, Merighi A, Bellis L, Scarcelli A, Manenti F: What is the utility of selected clinical and endoscopic parameters in predicting the risk of death after caustic ingestion? Endoscopy. 2002;34:304–10.

[51] Cheng YJ, Kao EL: Arterial blood gas analysis in acute caustic ingestion injuries. Surg Today. 2003;33:483–5.

[52] Thompson JN: Corrosive esophageal injuries. I. A study of nine cases of concurrent accidental caustic ingestion. Laryngoscope. 1987;97:1060–8.

[53] Doğan Y, Erkan T, Cokuğraş FC, Kutlu T: Caustic gastroesophageal lesions in childhood: an analysis of 473 cases. Clin Pediatr (Phila). 2006;45:435–8.

[54] Tiryaki T, Livanelioğlu Z, Atayurt H: Early bougienage for relief of stricture formation following caustic esophageal burns. Pediatr Surg Int. 2005;21:78–80.

[55] Iqbal CW, Askegard-Giesmann JR, Pham TH, Ishitani MB, Moir CR: Pediatric endoscopic injuries: incidence, management, and outcomes. J Pediatr Surg. 2008;43:911–5. doi: 10.1016/j.jpedsurg.2007.12.036.

[56] Gupta SK, Croffie JM, Fitzgerald JF: Is esophagogastroduodenoscopy necessary in all caustic ingestions? J Pediatr Gastroenterol Nutr. 2001;32:50–3.

[57] Millar AJ, Numanoglu A, Mann M, Marven S, Rode H: Detection of caustic oesophageal injury with technetium 99m-labelled sucralfate. J Pediatr Surg. 2001;36:262–5.

[58] Çiftçi ÖD, Gül SS, Açıksarı K, Maman A, Çavuşoğlu T, Bademci R, Taskiran D, Erbaş O: The diagnostic utility of scintigraphy in esophageal burn: a rat model. J Surg Res. 2016;200: 495–500. doi: 10.1016/j.jss.2015.09.006.

[59] Aksu B, Durmus-Altun G, Ustun F, Torun N, Kanter M, Umit H, Sut N: A new imaging modality in detection of caustic oesophageal injury: technetium-99m pyrophosphate scintigraphy. Int J Pediatr Otorhinolaryngol. 2009;73:409–15. doi:10.1016/j.ijporl.2008.11.008.

[60] Maurer AH, Parkman HP: Update on gastrointestinal scintigraphy. Semin Nucl Med. 2006;36:110–8.

[61] Warrington JC, Charron M: Pediatric gastrointestinal nuclear medicine. Semin Nucl Med. 2007;37:269–85.

[62] Kochhar R, Mittal BR, Kumar S, Bhattacharya A, Sethy PK, Dutta U: Segmental and total oesophageal transit time in patients with corrosive-induced oesophageal stricture. Nucl Med Commun. 2007;28:920–3.

[63] Kamijo Y, Kondo I, Soma K, Imaizumi H, Ohwada T: Alkaline esophagitis evaluated by endoscopic ultrasound. J Toxicol Clin Toxicol. 2001;39:623–5.

[64] Kamijo Y, Kondo I, Kokuto M, Kataoka Y, Soma K: Miniprobe ultrasonography for determining prognosis in corrosive esophagitis. Am J Gastroenterol. 2004;99:851–4.

[65] Kamijo Y, Kondo I, Watanabe M, Kan'o T, Ide A, Soma K: Gastric stenosis in severe corrosive gastritis: prognostic evaluation by endoscopic ultrasonography. Clin Toxicol (Phila). 2007;45:284–6.

[66] Chiu HM, Lin JT, Huang SP, Chen CH, Yang CS, Wang HP: Prediction of bleeding and stricture formation after corrosive ingestion by EUS concurrent with upper endoscopy. Gastrointest Endosc. 2004;60:827–33.

[67] Pelclová D, Navrátil T: Do corticosteroids prevent oesophageal stricture after corrosive ingestion? Toxicol Rev. 2005;24:125–9.

[68] Fulton JA, Hoffman RS: Steroids in second degree caustic burns of the esophagus: a systematic pooled analysis of fifty years of human data: 1956–2006. Clin Toxicol (Phila). 2007;45:402–8.

[69] Anderson KD, Rouse TM, Randolph JG: A controlled trial of corticosteroids in children with corrosive injury of the esophagus. N Engl J Med. 1990;323:637–40.

[70] Mamede RC, De Mello Filho FV: Treatment of caustic ingestion: an analysis of 239 cases. Dis Esophagus. 2002;15:210–3.

[71] Bautista A, Varela R, Villanueva A, Estevez E, Tojo R, Cadranel S: Effects of prednisolone and dexamethasone in children with alkali burns of the oesophagus. Eur J Pediatr Surg. 1996;6:198–203.

[72] Usta M, Erkan T, Cokugras FC, Urganci N, Onal Z, Gulcan M, Kutlu T: High doses of methylprednisolone in the management of caustic esophageal burns. Pediatrics. 2014;133:E1518–24.

[73] Boukthir S, Fetni I, Mrad SM, Mongalgi MA, Debbabi A, Barsaoui S: High doses of steroids in the management of caustic esophageal burns in children. Arch Pediatr. 2004;11:13–7.

[74] Andreoni B, Farina ML, Biffi R, Crosta C: Esophageal perforation and caustic injury: emergency management of caustic ingestion. Dis Esophagus. 1997;10:95–100.

[75] Cattan P, Munoz-Bongrand N, Berney T, Halimi B, Sarfati E, Celerier M: Extensive abdominal surgery after caustic ingestion. Ann Surg. 2000;231:519–23.

[76] Gün F, Abbasoğlu L, Celik A: Acute gastric perforation after acid ingestion. J Pediatr Gastroenterol Nutr. 2002;35:360–2.

[77] Ceylan H, Ozokutan BH, Gündüz F, Gözen A: Gastric perforation after corrosive ingestion. Pediatr Surg Int. 2011;27:649–53. doi:10.1007/s00383-010-2739-6.

[78] Boybeyi O, Karnak I, Tanyel FC, Senocak ME: Management of unusually extensive esophagogastric corrosive injuries: emergency measures and gastric reconstruction. J Pediatr Surg. 2009;44:1022–6. doi:10.1016/j.jpedsurg.2009.02.001.

[79] Uygun I, Arslan MS, Aydogdu B, Okur MH, Otcu S: Fluoroscopic balloon dilatation for caustic esophageal stricture in children: an 8-year experience. J Pediatr Surg. 2013;48:2230–4. doi:10.1016/j.jpedsurg.2013.04.005.

[80] Lan LC, Wong KK, Lin SC, Sprigg A, Clarke S, Johnson PR, Tam PK: Endoscopic balloon dilatation of esophageal strictures in infants and children: 17 years' experience and a literature review. J Pediatr Surg. 2003;38:1712–5.

[81] Pyrtle J, Obando J: Endoscopic management of difficult benign esophageal stricture. Tech Gastrointest Endosc. 2007;9:74–83.

[82] Poddar U, Thapa BR: Benign esophageal strictures in infants and children: results of Savary-Gilliard bougie dilation in 107 Indian children. Gastrointest Endosc. 2001;54:480–4.

[83] Kukkady A, Pease PW: Long-term dilatation of caustic strictures of the oesophagus. Pediatr Surg Int. 2002;18:486–90.

[84] Doo E-Y, Shin JH, Kim JH, Song H-Y: Oesophageal strictures caused by the ingestion of corrosive agents: effectiveness of balloon dilation in children. Clin Radiol. 2009; 64:265–71.

[85] Gündoğdu HZ, Tanyel FC, Büyükpamukçu N, Hiçsönmez A: Conservative treatment of caustic esophageal strictures in children. J Pediatr Surg. 1992;27:767–70.

[86] Alshammari J, Quesnel S, Pierrot S, Couloigner V: Endoscopic balloon dilatation of esophageal strictures in children. Int J Pediatr Otorhinolaryngol. 2011;75:1376–9. doi:10.1016/j.ijporl.2011.07.031.

[87] Vandenplas Y, Hauser B, Devreker T, Urbain D, Reynaert H: A biodegradable esophageal stent in the treatment of a corrosive esophageal stenosis in a child. J Pediatr Gastroenterol Nutr. 2009;49:254–7. doi: 10.1097/MPG.0b013e31819de871.

[88] Mutaf O: Treatment of corrosive esophageal strictures by long-term stenting. J Pediatr Surg. 1996;31:681–5.

[89] Chang CF, Kuo SP, Lin HC, Chuang CC, Tsai TK, Wu SF, Chen AC, Chen W, Peng CT: Endoscopic balloon dilatation for esophageal strictures in children younger than 6 years: experience in a medical center. Pediatr Neonatol. 2011;52:196–202. doi: 10.1016/j.pedneo.2011.05.005.

[90] Tam PKH, Sprigg A, Cudmore RE, Cook RC, Carty H: Endoscopy-guided balloon dilatation of esophageal strictures and anastomotic strictures after esophageal replacement in children. J Pediatr Surg. 1991;26:1101–3.

[91] Atabek C, Surer I, Demirbag S, Caliskan B, Ozturk H, Cetinkursun S: Increasing tendency in caustic esophageal burns and long-term polytetrafluorethylene stenting in severe cases: 10 years' experience. J Pediatr Surg. 2007;42:636–40.

[92] Foschia F, De Angelis P, Torroni F, Romeo E, Caldaro T, di Abriola GF, Pane A, Fiorenza MS, De Peppo F, Dall'Oglio L: Custom dynamic stent for esophageal strictures in children. J Pediatr Surg. 2011;46:848–53. doi: 10.1016/j.jpedsurg.2011.02.014.

[93] Zhang C, Zhou X, Yu L, Ding J, Shi R: Endoscopic therapy in the treatment of caustic esophageal stricture: a retrospective case series study. Dig Endosc. 2013;25:490–5. doi:10.1111/den.12023.

[94] Zhang C, Yu JM, Fan GP, Shi CR, Yu SY, Wang HP, Ge L, Zhong WX: The use of a retrievable self-expanding stent in treating childhood benign esophageal strictures. J Pediatr Surg. 2005;40:501–4.

[95] Heran MK, Baird R, Blair GK, Skarsgard ED: Topical mitomycin-C for recalcitrant esophageal strictures: a novel endoscopic/fluoroscopic technique for safe endoluminal delivery. J Pediatr Surg. 2008;43:815–8. doi: 10.1016/j.jpedsurg.2007.12.017.

[96] El-Asmar KM, Hassan MA, Abdelkader HM, Hamza AF: Topical mitomycin C can effectively alleviate dysphagia in children with long-segment caustic esophageal strictures. Dis Esophagus. 2015;28:422–7. doi: 10.1111/dote.12218.

[97] Kochhar R, Ray JD, Sriram PV, Kumar S, Singh K: Intralesional steroids augment the effects of endoscopic dilation in corrosive esophageal strictures. Gastrointest Endosc. 1999;49:509–13.

[98] El-Asmar KM, Hassan MA, Abdelkader HM, Hamza AF: Topical mitomycin C application is effective in management of localized caustic esophageal stricture: a double-blinded, randomized, placebo-controlled trial. J Pediatr Surg. 2013;48:1621–7. doi: 10.1016/j.jpedsurg.2013.04.014.

[99] Heran MK, Pham TH, Butterworth S, Robinson A: Use of a microporous polytetrafluoroethylene catheter balloon to treat refractory esophageal stricture: a novel technique for delivery of mitomycin C. J Pediatr Surg. 2011;46:776–9. doi: 10.1016/j.jpedsurg.2010.11.030.

[100] Hamza AF, Abdelhay S, Sherif H, Hasan T, Soliman H, Kabesh A, Bassiouny I, Bahnassy AF: Caustic esophageal strictures in children: 30 years' experience. J Pediatr Surg. 2003;38:828–33.

[101] Angotti R, Molinaro F, Noviello C, Cobellis G, Martino A, Del Rossi C, Bianchi A, Messina M: Gastric transposition as a valid surgical option for esophageal replacement in pediatric patients: experience from three Italian medical centers. Gastroenterol Rep (Oxf). 2016;pii: gow012:1–5. doi:10.1093/gastro/gow012.

[102] Arul GS, Parikh D: Oesophageal replacement in children. Ann R Coll Surg Engl. 2008;90:7–12. doi: 10.1308/003588408X242222.

[103] Spitz L, Kiely E, Pierro A: Gastric transposition in children—a 21-year experience. J Pediatr Surg. 2004;39:276–81; discussion 276–81.

[104] Spitz L: Esophageal replacement: overcoming the need. J Pediatr Surg. 2014;49:849–52. doi: 10.1016/j.jpedsurg.2014.01.011.

[105] Gündoğdu HZ, Tanyel FC, Büyükpamukçu N, Hiçsönmez A: Colonic replacement for the treatment of caustic esophageal strictures in children. J Pediatr Surg. 1992;27:771–4.

[106] Ezemba N, Eze JC, Nwafor IA, Etukokwu KC, Orakwe OI: Colon interposition graft for corrosive esophageal stricture: midterm functional outcome. World J Surg. 2014;38:2352–7. doi: 10.1007/s00268-014-2574-3.

[107] Ergün O, Celik A, Mutaf O: Two-stage coloesophagoplasty in children with caustic burns of the esophagus: hemodynamic basis of delayed cervical anastomosis—theory and fact. J Pediatr Surg. 2004;39:545–8.

[108] Bothereau H, Munoz-Bongrand N, Lambert B, Montemagno S, Cattan P, Sarfati E: Esophageal reconstruction after caustic injury: is there still a place for right coloplasty? Am J Surg. 2007;193:660–4.

[109] Coopman S, Michaud L, Halna-Tamine M, Bonnevalle M, Bourgois B, Turck D, Gottrand F: Long-term outcome of colon interposition after esophagectomy in children. J Pediatr Gastroenterol Nutr. 2008;47:458–62. doi: 10.1097/MPG.0b013e31815ce55c.

[110] Boukerrouche A: Left colonic graft in esophageal reconstruction for caustic stricture: mortality and morbidity. Dis Esophagus. 2013;26:788–93. doi: 10.1111/j.1442-2050.2012.01383.x.

[111] Boukerrouche A: Isoperistaltic left colic graft interposition via a retrosternal approach for esophageal reconstruction in patients with a caustic stricture: mortality, morbidity, and functional results. Surg Today. 2014;44:827–33. doi: 10.1007/s00595-013-0758-3.

[112] Raffensperger JG, Luck SR, Reynolds M, Schwartz D: Intestinal bypass of the esophagus. J Pediatr Surg. 1996;31:38–46; discussion 46–7.

[113] Chirica M, Veyrie N, Munoz-Bongrand N, Zohar S, Halimi B, Celerier M, Cattan P, Sarfati E: Late morbidity after colon interposition for corrosive esophageal injury: risk factors, management, and outcome. A 20-years' experience. Ann Surg. 2010;252:271–80. doi: 10.1097/SLA.0b013e3181e8fd40.

[114] Spitz L: Gastric transposition in children. Semin Pediatr Surg. 2009;18:30–3. doi: 10.1053/j.sempedsurg.2008.10.006.

[115] Marujo WC, Tannuri U, Maksoud JG: Total gastric transposition: an alternative to esophageal replacement in children. J Pediatr Surg. 1991;26:676–81.

[116] Davenport M, Hosie GP, Tasker RC, Gordon I, Kiely EM, Spitz L: Long-term effects of gastric transposition in children: a physiological study. J Pediatr Surg. 1996;31:588–93.

[117] Tannuri U, Maksoud-Filho JG, Tannuri AC, Andrade W, Maksoud JG: Which is better for esophageal substitution in children, esophagocoloplasty or gastric transposition? A 27-year experience of a single center. J Pediatr Surg. 2007;42:500–4.

[118] Dehghani SM, Aldaghi M, Javaherizadeh H: Endoscopic pyloroplasty for severe gastric outlet obstruction due to alkali ingestion in a child. Gastroenterol Hepatol Bed Bench. 2016;9:64–7.

[119] Temiz A, Oguzkurt P, Ezer SS, Ince E, Gezer HO, Hicsonmez A: Management of pyloric stricture in children: endoscopic balloon dilatation and surgery. Surg Endosc. 2012;26:1903–8. doi: 10.1007/s00464-011-2124-0.

[120] Ozokutan BH, Ceylan H, Ertaşkin I, Yapici S: Pediatric gastric outlet obstruction following corrosive ingestion. Pediatr Surg Int. 2010;26:615–8. doi: 10.1007/s00383-010-2613-6.

[121] Chaudhary A, Puri AS, Dhar P, Reddy P, Sachdev A, Lahoti D, Kumar N, Broor SL: Elective surgery for corrosive induced gastric injury. World J Surg. 1996;20:703–6

[122] Mutaf O, Genç A, Herek O, Demircan M, Ozcan C, Arikan A: Gastroesophageal reflux: a determinant in the outcome of caustic esophageal burns. J Pediatr Surg. 1996; 31:1494–5.